ALCOHOL, DISABILITIES, AND REHABILITATION

ALCOHOL, DISABILITIES, AND REHABILITATION

Susan A. Storti, R.N., M.A., C.D.N.S., C.A.S.

Brown University
Center for Alcohol and Addiction Studies
Providence, Rhode Island

SINGULAR PUBLISHING GROUP, INC.
SAN DIEGO · LONDON

Singular Publishing Group, Inc.
401 West "A" Street, Suite 325
San Diego, California 92101-7904

Singular Publishing Ltd.
19 Compton Terrace
London N1 2UN, U.K.

e-mail: singpub@mail.cerfnet.com
Web site: http://www.singpub.com

Typeset in 10/12 Bookman by SoCal Graphics
Printed in United States of America by McNaughton and Gunn

Library of Congress Cataloging-in-Publication Data

Storti, Susan A.
Alcohol, disabilities, and rehabilitation / Susan A. Storti.
p. cm
Includes bibliographical references and index.
ISBN 1-56593-690-6
1. Alcoholism—Treatment. 2. Alcoholics—Rehabilitation
I. Title.
RC565.S748 1997
616.86'1—dc21 97-12959
CIP

CONTENTS

FOREWORD

This book provides an exciting bridge between two significant arenas: Alcohol problems and the rehabilitation of those with chronic illness. As this book details, alcohol and alcohol problems occur frequently and have significant effects on the etiology, course, and prognosis of medical conditions. You can't work clinically without being struck by the ability of alcohol to permeate and affect so many people, diagnoses, treatments, etc. The magnitude of the problem can be overwhelming. All of us who work in the health and other professional care fields are keenly aware that the more we know and have experience within an area, the more effective we can be in our care, assistance, and interventions. Until now the dilemma was how to keep abreast of all you need to know about alcohol—its effects, assessment, and treatment—let alone integrate it all within our particular clinical work. This book addresses that gap. It provides those of us in rehabilitation, medical, and related fields with solid information about alcohol and its effects as well as practical assessment and intervention strategies.

One of the great rewards of teaching is that you often learn more from your students than you are able to convey to them. I first met Sue Storti when she was completing her master's degree in Rehabilitation Counseling. This book conveys the best of what struck me then. Here is someone with a background in nursing, an excellent grasp of chronic medical conditions, and a vast knowledge, background, and experience in alcohol and substance abuse. But most importantly Sue Storti articulates the issues, discusses the concepts, and suggests sensible pragmatic interventions. All of us, nurses, therapists, social workers, physicians, and others, learned a lot during her stay on the rehabilitation ward and outpatient service.

This book continues and goes beyond that experience. Whether reading about background concepts and knowledge, the relationship of alcohol to medically related issues, assessment, or interventions I was repeatedly excited by new information and material that had a direct bearing on my clinical work. The writing is clear, the content cutting edge, and the clinical suggestions straightforward. This is a book for nursing stations, wards, nursing homes, and clinical offices. It's a great education read cover to cover but equally solid as a quick reference and guide. As such it will appeal to academicians and clinicians alike.

Duane S. Bishop, M.D.

PREFACE

Despite growing evidence of the serious and persisting consequences of alcohol misuse and abuse, we all behave, at times, in ways that could lead to alcohol dependency under the right circumstances. Given that we all engage in such behaviors to some extent, the issue becomes one of understanding why some of us become alcohol dependent, while others are mildly affected.

The range of severity of alcohol use and abuse in patients who are hospitalized secondary to physical injury is quite heterogeneous. These patients present a special challenge to health care professionals trying to respond to their unique needs. Accordingly, this calls for creativity on the part of the rehabilitation staff who are attempting to meet the needs of injured and/or disabled alcohol abusing patients. To effectively respond to this challenge, health care providers need to develop a foundation of knowledge in the area of alcohol use, abuse, and dependency. It is this need that is the focus of this book.

A key issue facing health care providers today is determining for whom and under what circumstances, which type of intervention is most likely to be effective. Several decades of research and clinical experience indicate the many and diverse problems associated with alcohol misuse and alcoholism demand a range of treatment approaches to meet patient needs.

This book offers a broad selection of information about alcohol. Included among the subject areas are the relationship between alcohol and trauma; the psychological, physiological, and social consequences of the abuse of alcohol on individuals and the family unit; tools for screening and assessment; and an overview of traditional and emerging treatment approaches. It has been written in a clear concise style suitable for use by all, from concerned family members to addiction specialists.

Its contents will serve as a resource for individuals such as health care and allied health care providers, students, substance abuse prevention and treatment professionals, and rehabilitation specialists, to name a few. Community-based agencies and other health-related organizations may also find it of assistance in educating staff and enhancing service delivery.

This publication is written with hope that you will gain an understanding and a greater awareness of the potential problems associated with alcohol misuse, abuse, and alcoholism.

ACKNOWLEDGMENTS

I would like to acknowledge my family, friends, and colleagues who have contributed to this effort over the past three years. Through your continuous encouragement and support, this book evolved from a concept to a reality. Thank you.

CHAPTER 1

ALCOHOL AND INJURIES:

What's the Connection?

- **Alcohol and the Disabled Population**
- **Epidemiology of Alcohol-Related Trauma**
- **Types of Injuries**

For many years we have known that alcohol and other drugs are major precipitants of physical injury. In addition, we also know that physically challenged individuals are at higher risk for developing chemical dependency. The litany of drug-related problems and damage to persons and society seems endless. Damaged health, injury, and death result. In recent years there has been a growing awareness that many problems encountered by human service professionals are either a direct result of or at least complicated by an addiction of one form or another. Single episodes of drinking or drug use, persistent substance abuse, and substance dependence can result in a variety of adverse social consequences that can affect a host of people ranging from an individual to society as a whole.

In the United States, injuries are the leading cause of death among persons younger than age 44 and the leading cause of life years lost because of premature death (Harrington, Putnam, Waters, & Colt, 1989; National Center for Injury Prevention and Control, 1991). Each year, more than 2 million persons are injured seriously enough to be hospitalized, and more than 80,000 Americans receive permanently disabling injuries to the brain and spinal cord. For each death resulting from injury, 19 other injured persons are hospitalized and 354 receive medical care (Adams & Benson, 1993).

ALCOHOL AND THE DISABLED POPULATION

The issue of alcohol, tobacco, and other drug (ATOD) problems among individuals with disabilities emerged when it became increasingly apparent that the incidence of ATOD problems among people with certain disabilities was above the national average for the general population, which is estimated at 10 to 12%. Studies indicate that the rate of ATOD problems among individuals with disabilities may range from 15 to 30% (Buss & Cramer, 1989; deMiranda & Cherry, 1989).

Although people with disabilities, whether the disability is a result of a traumatic injury or is an existing condition, are at a greater risk of having ATOD-related problems, these problems often go unrecognized and unaddressed for various reasons. People with disabilities are likely to deny, hide, or discount ATOD problems in order to escape the "double negative" of being socially stigmatized with both disability and ATOD-related problems. A poor self-concept or self-esteem may keep a person with a disability from seeking help or from recognizing the potential for recovery. More practically, the limited financial resources of most people with disabilities may prohibit treatment.

Historically, rehabilitation professionals have failed to address the link between ATOD problems and disability. There are a number of interrelated reasons for this failure, including lack of preservice training or accreditation standards, lack of interdisciplinary training, labeling an ATOD problem as a "secondary disability," and gaps in the system that perpetuate a sense that ATOD problems are someone else's problem.

Whatever the causes, there are severe consequences for ignoring the relationship between ATOD problems and disability. Over $25 billion is spent annually in the United States on direct and indirect costs of medical, rehabilitative, and support services, and lost productivity in the workplace. Lifetime costs for a serious disability can run to $9 million. ATOD problems can undermine rehabilitation efforts and aggravate chronic health conditions, thus increasing associated ongoing health care and related costs. Intervening to prevent and address ATOD problems can significantly improve outcomes for people with disabilities, and curb associated medical and rehabilitation costs.

EPIDEMIOLOGY OF ALCOHOL-RELATED TRAUMA

Trauma is the leading cause of death attributable to the use of ATODs and a major public health problem. Trauma is usually caused by motor vehicle crashes, suicide and homicide, falls, burns, or drowning. Injuries may be fatal or nonfatal and may result in death or temporary, partial, or permanent disability.

Alcohol has many physical and psychological effects that contribute to traumatic injuries. These include decreased level of alertness, impairment of motor function, diminishment of coordination and balance, increase in reaction time, impairment of judgment, impairment of perception and cognitive abilities, increase in risk taking behaviors and feelings of invulnerability, increased violent behavior, an effect on emotions and reduction in inhibitions, intensification of feelings of anger and depression, and an increase in impulsive behaviors. In addition, chronic alcohol use can render an individual more medically fragile, and thus injuries sustained are more severe.

Extensive research has linked alcohol abuse with the occurrence of traumatic injury (Baker, O'Neill, Ginsburg, & Li, 1992; Lowenfels & Miller, 1984; National Academy of Sciences, 1985; Smith & Krauss, 1988; Soderstrom, 1989). According to Lowenfels and Miller (1984), alcohol intoxication is associated with 40 to 50% of traffic fatalities; 25 to 35% of nonfatal motor vehicle injuries; 9 to 86% of fires, burns, and burn fatalities (Combs-Orme, Taylor, Scott, & Holmes, 1983; Howland & Hingson, 1987; Schmidt & deLint, 1972); 48% of hypothermia and frostbite cases; 41% of drownings (Roizen, 1982); and approximately 20% of completed suicides. The prevalent evidence linking alcohol to recreational accidents, including boats and aquatic sports, suggests that the use of alcohol has been a significant factor in drownings that result when individuals inadvertently fall into the water (Dietz & Baker, 1974). Alcohol has also been estimated to be present in 40% or more of falls and nearly 50% of homicides (victims or perpetrator). The use and abuse of alcohol has been identified as the single most important human factor associated with fatal injuries (Harrington et al., 1989).

Research has also found that many alcoholic patients have experienced trauma in the early stages of their problem drinking, and a history of trauma in hospitalized patients with an injury has been found to be an indicator of alcohol abuse and alcoholism (Cesare, Morgan, Felice, & Edge, 1990; Clark, McCarthy, & Robinson, 1985; Maull, Clapp, & Ellis, 1986; Skinner, Holt, Schuller, Roy, & Israell, 1984; Swan, 1989). In addition, alcoholism has been found to be the most common chronic illness found in trauma patients, affecting as many as one fourth of victims requiring hospital care for their injuries (Antti-Poika, 1986; Antti-Poika, Karaharju, Roine, & Salaspuro, 1988; Maull, 1982; Rivara, Koepsell, Jurkovich, Gurney, & Soderberg, 1993).

Alcohol's association with trauma was recognized and documented long ago. A passage in an Egyptian papyrus dated 1500 B.C. warns that excessive drinking can lead to falls and broken bones (el-Guebaly & el-Guebaly, 1981). The scientific investigation of alcohol's relationship to injury has been under way for nearly a century; the short-term physiological effects of alcohol include diminished motor coordination and balance, along with impairment of attention, perception, and judgment regarding behavior. Such effects may place the drinker at higher risk for alcohol-related injuries (Fell, 1992). Alcohol use may be involved directly in an injury event and may be associated with behaviors that increase the risk for injury. Alcohol users increase their risk in two ways: likelihood of injury and seriousness of injury. First, alcohol abusers are more likely than sober persons to be involved in a traumatic event, and second, given similar traumatic circumstances, research suggests that alcohol may render an individual more vulnerable to injury in the event of trauma (French, 1991; National Institute on Alcohol Abuse and Alcoholism, 1989; Redfern, Rees, & Owen, 1988; Roizen, 1988; Waller, Hansen, & Stewart, 1989).

It is also important to note that alcohol frequently complicates diagnosis of trauma-related injury (Lowenfels & Miller,

1984; Soderstrom, DuPriest, Benner, Maekawa, & Cowley, 1979). Alcoholics who incur trauma present a special dilemma. Because of their tolerance, they may show no evidence of intoxication, resulting in a variety of unexpected alcohol-related complications arising during trauma management. For example, many alcoholics vary in their response to therapeutic drugs, depending on the recency of their last drink. An alcoholic patient may enter withdrawal, further complicating management of the traumatic event; or the signs of intoxication that the patient exhibits can mimic other conditions, causing overdiagnosis, as in the case of a serious head injury.

Alcohol use and the impairment that results from it has also been empirically linked to spinal cord injury (SCI) and traumatic brain injury (TBI). For people with TBI and SCI, abuse of alcohol often precedes the disability and is among its causes. Emergency room rates of major trauma, including SCI, show intoxication rates of 39–50% (Heinemann, 1991). In more than half of all cases involving persons who incur TBI, alcohol abuse has been indicated; the percentage can range up to 72% in some groups of patients (Sparadeo & Gill, 1989). If the disability is a direct result of alcohol use, or if it predates the disability, the chances are greater that the problems will continue following rehabilitation.

In addition, alcohol has been associated with cardiac arrhythmias, cardiomyopathy, and hypertension, all predisposing factors to cerebral vascular accidents (CVAs) or strokes. Abuse of alcohol reduces the cerebral blood flow (CBF), which can produce ischemia in the brain, resulting in stroke. According to Altura and Altura (1990), when compared with nondrinkers, light drinkers have almost double the risk of experiencing hemorrhagic stroke syndrome and heavy drinkers have almost triple the risk.

The accumulated evidence makes it very clear that health care professionals who treat injured persons with high blood alcohol concentrations (BAC) need to address the problem themselves, if possible, or refer these individuals to rehabilitation for further evaluation of their drinking patterns (Lowenstein, Weissberg, & Terry, 1990).

It is important to note that research has documented that individuals who have sustained one traumatic injury are at an increased risk of reinjury. Many clinicians, researchers, and epidemiologists believe that rates of readmission for second and third traumatic injuries are strongly related to untreated substance use problems (Meyers, Zepeda, & Murdock, 1990; Rivara et al., 1993). For example, after one head injury a person is three times more likely than someone in the general population to sustain a second head injury. After a second injury, the relative risk for a third injury increases to eight times the normal risk (Annegers, Grabow, Kurland, & Laws, 1980).

The available literature concerning the involvement of alcohol and other drugs in unintentional injuries has led the Centers for Disease Control and Prevention to urge health care providers in emergency rooms to consider increasing testing of injured patients for alcohol and other drugs, to both ensure appropriate medical management of injuries and serve as the first step in treating alcohol and other drug use and dependency problems.

TYPES OF INJURIES

As previously stated, traumatic injuries are often related to the use of alcohol and/or other drugs. Traumatic brain injury, spinal cord injury, and stroke are the most devastating types of injury because they often result in permanent loss of function.

Traumatic Brain Injury

Traumatic brain injury (TBI) refers to damage to the brain caused by external mechanical forces applied to the head. TBI may produce a diminished or altered state of consciousness, ranging from slight dizziness to coma. It may result in impairment of cognitive abilities and/or physical, emotional, and behavioral functioning. It is acquired suddenly and typically results in brain damage that is diffuse, affecting the whole brain and brain stem. Thus, impairments are multiple and many aspects of life are changed.

Physical disabilities resulting from head injury range from minimal motor deficits to complete paralysis, and may either be temporary or permanent. Even patients with mild head injuries can experience devastating effects in their long-term recovery from injury. Cognitive disabilities may include impairments in executive function (problem solving, abstraction, impulse control, and judgment), orientation, attention, and concentration, learning and memory, language, visuoperceptual function (spatial relationships), reasoning, and general intelligence. Other effects can include insomnia and vertigo.

Many head-injured patients need extensive rehabilitation for serious cognitive deficits caused by the injury. Health care professionals who encounter these patients may be baffled by their impulsivity and impaired memory and may become frustrated about the compliance problems these patients have with any type of treatment, including alcohol dependency treatment.

Spinal Cord Injuries

Spinal cord injury (SCI) is a lesion that may involve complete or incomplete disruption of the spinal cord. The causes of SCIs are similar to those of TBI, and the two injuries can occur as a result of the same event. SCIs can result in permanent motor disability, usually paraplegia or quadriplegia, and varying degrees of motor and sensory deficits. Postinjury, some body organs may require retraining and daily management.

Approximately 50% of spinal cord injuries are due to motor vehicle and motorcycle crashes; falls account for approximately 20% of these injuries; and approximately 15% are attributed to drug and alcohol related violence (Kraus, 1992; Stover & Fine, 1986).

Stroke

Stroke, also referred to as a *cerebral vascular accident*, is the third leading cause of death in the United States among adults and is a major cause of disability in the elderly. Stroke is defined as any condition during which blood supply to the brain is interrupted, resulting in loss of consciousness, paralysis, or other symptoms, depending on the site and extent of brain damage. The types of strokes are further divided into *hemorrhagic* strokes or *ischemic* strokes, and by the area of the brain affected (*subarachnoid* stroke or *intracerebral* stroke).

A stroke is not an accident as the term cerebral vascular accident suggests. Instead, the development of *atherosclerosis* and the occurrence of a stroke are related to a number of risk factors (Gorelick & Kelly, 1992), which include age, gender, familial factors, diabetes mellitus, prior stroke, asymptomatic carotid bruits, hypertension, cardiac disease, transient ischemic attacks, elevated hematocrit, sickle cell disease, serum cholesterol, glucose intolerance, cigarette smoking, left ventricular hypertrophy, body weight, and parental death (Dyken et al., 1984; Paffenbarger & Williams, 1967; Wolf, Kannel, & Verter, 1983).

Alcohol was recognized as a possible risk factor for stroke as early as 1725 (Gorelick, 1989). The association was not emphasized again until the 1950s and 1960s, when alcohol was thought to predispose young adults to ischemic stroke. In the 1970s and early 1980s, a series of published articles linked ischemic brain infarction in young adults and adolescents with occasional ethanol intoxication, and in middle-aged women and young men with both occasional alcohol intoxication and regular heavy drinking (Gorelick & Kelly, 1992).

Alcohol has been shown to increase the risk for hypertension, cardiomyopathy, sudden death, and hemorrhagic stroke. The physiological mechanisms by which alcohol predisposes a person to ischemic stroke include disorders of the cardiovascular system, such as "holiday heart" syndrome (Gorelick, 1990), coagulation and platelet disorders, and cerebral blood flow and metabolism (Gorelick, 1989; NIAAA, 1994).

Strokes of all types are major contributors to disability, and when severe, treatment usually fails to restore the patient to the prestroke state. These patients require extensive rehabilitative therapy, and clinicians often need to develop innovative treatment strategies to address alcohol-related issues in this patient population.

Internal Injuries

Internal injuries include blunt and penetrating injuries to internal organs and are often multiple. Causes of internal injuries include motor vehicle, motorcycle, and bicycle crashes, falls, sports, and violence. Injuries resulting from motor vehicle crashes and violence, especially stabbings, have a well documented relationship with alcohol and other drugs.

SUMMARY

These are just a few examples of how the use of alcohol can disrupt and destroy the lives of persons who drink as well as the innocent persons who fall victim to the ramifications of alcoholism.

Very often, a history of alcohol abuse and/or dependency is identified among individuals who are physically disabled secondary to a traumatic injury. It has been reported that at least 60% of medical-surgical and SCI patients have alcohol as a complicating factor of the primary medical illness for which they were admitted to the hospital (Mourer, 1992).

In the past, individuals suffering from alcoholism were seen as individuals who suffered from a sociopathic illness. Today, health care providers have a better understanding of the disease of addiction and have come to realize that a large number of the people they care for suffer from alcohol abuse or alcoholism. Often, these patients are remembered because of the difficulty and frustration they present to the professionals trying to serve them.

CHAPTER 2

OVERVIEW OF PSYCHOACTIVE SUBSTANCE USE, ABUSE, AND DEPENDENCY

- **Terminology and Key Concepts**
- **Phenomena of Addiction**

To prevent and treat alcohol-related consequences, some basic terminology and concepts must be understood. Toward that end, a compendium of terms and concepts as they relate to alcohol are presented in this chapter. To begin, let us first define the term *drug*.

TERMINOLOGY AND KEY CONCEPTS

A *drug* is defined as any substance, natural or artificial, other than body constituents or those needed for normal body functioning that has a psychoactive, chemical, or medicinal effect when ingested (Ray & Ksir, 1993). Although alcohol is considered to be a "drug," for the purposes of this book its abuse is discussed separately from that of other drugs.

A *drug of abuse* is any substance that alters mood, level of perception, or brain functioning. These substances include prescribed medications, alcohol, solvents, and illegal drugs (Schuckit, 1989). A *psychoactive* or mood-altering substance changes a person's mood and/or behavior (Ray & Ksir, 1993; Schnoll, 1986). Some are legal substances and have been approved for sale either by prescription or over the counter. Others are illegal substances whose manufacture, sale, purchasing for sale, or possession is prohibited. These substances may also include federally approved drugs that are obtained by illegal means or used for illicit purposes.

What Is Alcohol?

Alcohol is a central nervous system depressant. At high blood levels, alcohol leads to respiratory depression, respiratory arrest, and death. At low blood levels, alcohol impairs regulatory and inhibitory control mechanisms in the brain. Complex and learned behaviors are impaired. Individuals often become generally disinhibited and engage in high risk sexual behaviors that could put them at risk for contracting the human immunodeficiency virus (Cooper, 1992). Anxiety is reduced; judgment is poor; and attention, short-term memory, and thought processing are impaired. As blood levels rise, motor coordination becomes impaired, and reaction time becomes quite prolonged. If drinking continues, stupor, coma, and death can ensue.

The *stimulant* drugs, such as amphetamines, cocaine, and caffeine, excite the nervous system which leads to increased alertness, a sense of well-being, and behavioral activities. At higher doses, they can produce a manic state of excitement combined with paranoia and hallucinations. The *depressant* drugs (e.g., alcohol, benzodiazepines, sedative-hypnotics, inhalants) inhibit central nervous system activity resulting in decreased anxiety levels, slowed reaction times, uncoordinated movements, and in higher doses, sleep. The third category of drugs, *narcotics* (e.g., opium, heroin), are a group of analgesic drugs that produce a relaxed, dreamlike state. At high doses, they can also induce sleep. The *hallucinogens* (e.g., LSD and *phencyclidine* or

PCP) can produce visual and auditory hallucinations and an altered sense of reality. The final category of drugs, *psychotherapeutics*, includes a variety of drugs prescribed for the control of mental illness. The *antipsychotics*, sometimes referred to as major tranquilizers, help to control hallucinations and illogical thoughts. The *antidepressants*, such as lithium, help to control depressed mood states.

In most classification systems some things do not fit into any one category. For example, marijuana is sometimes included in the category of hallucinogens; however, more often than not, it stands alone. The reason is that marijuana can produce sedative effects like depressants, but in large doses, it can produce hallucinogenic effects. As a result of its unique properties, it is often placed on its own. Another example is nicotine, which is often considered a stimulant; however, it also has some relaxant effects like a depressant.

Key Concepts

Throughout this text a variety of terms will be used frequently to describe the problem of dependency and those who are affected by it. To avoid misinterpretation, several of these terms are described here.

Substance abuse. The concept of substance abuse is fairly simple. It is taken to mean the unauthorized use of mood-altering drugs, frequently in amounts that interfere with an individual's physical, occupational, psychological, or social functioning (Mattox, 1986). Thus, whether or when an individual's chemical use is either appropriate or abusive depends on acceptable social and medical standards and on cultural and personal values.

Drug of Choice. In this era of polydrug addiction, the concept of drug of choice is very important. It is best described in the form of a question: Of all the possible drugs available, including any and all drugs the individual may have used in the past, what specific drug, or drugs, would this individual use if given his or her choice? For example, many cocaine addicts will use alcohol to help control the side effects of cocaine. The use of alcohol is secondary to their drug of choice, which is cocaine (Doweiko, 1993).

Addiction. Despite repeated efforts to define it, the concept of addiction remains poorly distinguished from that of habit and is used loosely in describing any compulsion. It has been applied in popular discussion in the media and often in professional and research literature in a vague way to a wide range of behaviors. Since alcohol use may or may not lead to addiction and definitions vary, the term *dependence* is now often used as an alternative to, or interchangeably with, addiction.

The concept of dependency goes beyond the physical effects of alcohol on the body to encompass its behavioral aspects. In the context of this book, *alcohol dependency* refers to a state of periodic or chronic intoxication, as a result of a loss of control and the continued use of alcohol despite adverse consequences. It is characterized by an overpowering preoccupation with and compulsion to obtain and consume alcohol, a need to increase the amount of alcohol consumed, and the presentation of withdrawal symptoms on cessation of drinking (Ray & Ksir, 1993; Schnoll, 1986). Chemical dependency, which includes alcohol, includes a psychological and/or physiological dependence.

Tolerance refers to the body's physiological adaptation to the toxic effects of a drug, hence the need to increase the dosage of the drug to achieve the desired response (Portenoy & Payne, 1992). Schuckit (1989) identifies two forms of tolerance to a drug: metabolic tolerance and pharmacodynamic tolerance.

Metabolic tolerance takes place when the liver becomes more efficient at metabolizing alcohol as a result of continuous exposure. This increase in metabolism causes a more rapid elimination from the blood. *Pharmacodynamic tolerance* is a term that describes the increasing insensitivity of the central nervous system to alcohol's effects. When the cells of the central nervous system are continuously exposed to a chemical, the cells will adapt to maintain normal functioning by making minute changes in their structure. These cells then become less sensitive to the effects of the chemical to achieve the desired response. The body begins to require periodic doses of the drug to function normally and to maintain physiological homeostasis.

When there is a sudden or gradual cessation of the use of a drug, such as alcohol, a characteristic withdrawal *syndrome* will result. The exact nature of the syndrome will depend on a variety of factors, such as the length of time that alcohol has been abused, the amount consumed, and the individual's state of health.

Withdrawal is usually accompanied by physical symptoms that are specific to each group of drugs. The withdrawal syndrome may consist of an acute and a prolonged stage. The acute stage usually lasts 2 to 7 days, with the most pronounced withdrawal symptoms present during this period. The prolonged stage, or *protracted abstinence syndrome*, may last for weeks or months and is less intense. It is believed that these protracted symptoms may make a person more vulnerable to relapse.

The existence of a withdrawal syndrome is evidence that a *physiological dependence* has developed. This withdrawal syndrome is the direct result of the absence of the chemical that caused cellular adaptation, in this case, alcohol. When the alcohol is discontinued, the central nervous system must readapt to again function normally without its presence. It is during this readaptation period that the physical signs of withdrawal are present. It is important to state that physiological dependence occurs with some drugs and not with others, and this physiological adaptation that plays a key role in the development of alcohol dependency.

Psychological dependence refers to the psychosocial adaptation and craving for a drug. The term *habituation* has been applied to this phenomenon as well. The person believes the substance to be necessary to maintain well-being, and the preoccupation with the drug's effect may be so central to the person's existence that it becomes a craving or compulsion. The greater the reliance on or perceived benefit of a drug, the more efforts made to get it. Psychological dependence may develop with or without the physical adaptation by the body to the use of the drugs. The psychological aspects of dependency are as critical as, or more critical than, the physical dependence and may dominate life to the exclusion of all else.

In the context of dependency, it is also important to understand the concepts of abstinence and relapse. *Abstinence* refers to refraining from the use of alcohol (Ray & Ksir, 1993), and *relapse* refers to the return to use after a period of abstinence (Schnoll, 1986).

The final two concepts of significance are *cross tolerance* and *cross dependence.* Certain drugs with similar properties are cross-tolerant with each other, indicating the development of tolerance to all drugs within a class. For example, the alcoholic will demonstrate tolerance to other sedative-hypnotic drugs.

Cross-dependence implies that one drug can prevent the withdrawal syndrome when another drug on which the person is physiologically dependent is withheld.

PHENOMENA OF ADDICTION

In the previous sections an introduction to the basic terminology and key concepts as they relate to dependency were provided. Let us now explore how an individual who uses drugs progresses along the continuum of use from experimentation to dependency (Figure 2–1). The process of addiction occurs in stages that progress in varying time frames depending on the individual, the substance, and the risk factors involved. It is important to note that the progression is not always a linear movement in one direction. The individual may remain in one stage or move between stages for a period of time.

There are a variety of patterns ranging from *experimentation* to dependency. As we begin to examine the process, we must first acknowledge the individual whose behavior is reflective of total abstinence. This individual abstains from any and all recreational alcohol and chemical use (Akers, 1992).

As we move from left to right on the continuum, we enter into the first stage, referred to as experimentation. At this stage, the individual feels he or she has the ability and control to drink

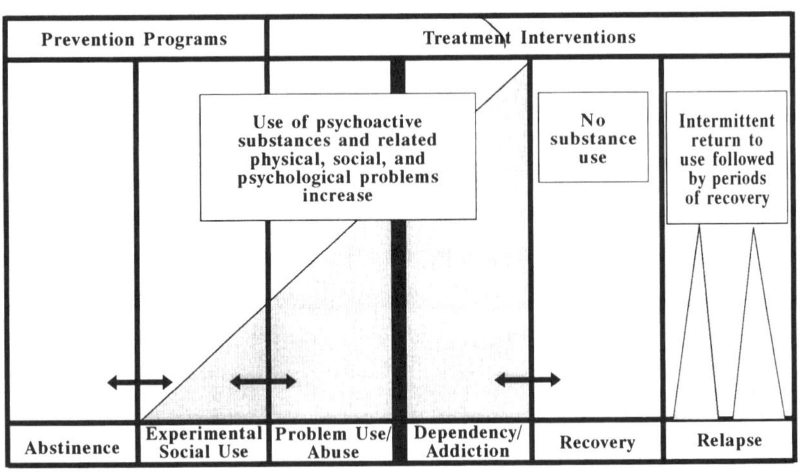

FIGURE 2–1. The Process of Addiction. (From Treatment for Alcohol and Other Drug Abuse—Opportunities for Coordination, by A. H. Crowe & R. Reeves, 1994, (Technical Assistance Publication [TAP] Series 11, DHHS Publication No. SMA 94-2075), p. 5. Copyright by the U.S. Department of Health and Human Services.)

or take a drug a few times and then stop. The fact is, many can do this; however, many cannot. This initial contact with psychoactive substances usually occurs during the adolescent years, and may occur in a social setting or as a result of the use of a substance prescribed for medical purposes. As use continues, other illicit drugs may be consumed. During this initial period, use of drugs is intermittent, and most people return to a period of complete abstinence during which they do not seek or consume drugs and experience no adverse consequences (Institute of Medicine, 1990b; Naegle, 1993).

It is important to understand that psychoactive drugs mimic, displace, block, or deplete specific chemical messengers between nerve cells in the brain. As a result they produce a rewarding mental state (e.g., euphoria), which functions as positive reinforcer on use. Thus, continued exposure to alcohol and other drugs can initiate increased drug-seeking behavior and set the stage for addiction (Dackis & Gold, 1992; Institute of Medicine, 1990b).

Having enjoyed the effects of the drug, individuals begin to use drugs more frequently. This stage, referred to as *occasional* use, varies in length of time and intensity. For some, occasional use stops after a period of time. But for others, this reinforcing experience may lead to an increase in drug or alcohol consumption. These individuals may begin to use in a *regular pattern*—such as weekend parties and with friends. Some people stay at this stage and do not progress any further. But for others, alcohol and/or drug use becomes a way to overcome shyness, relieve boredom, deal with loneliness, or as an escape from responsibilities.

The next stage is referred to as *abuse*, and is marked by an increase in frequency and amount of alcohol consumed or the drug used. Use to the point of intoxication often occurs. The pleasurable, euphoric feelings produced with earlier use are still sought, but after the effects of the drug subside, pain, depression, and discomfort occur. Unlike earlier stages of use, individuals progressing through this stage are likely to begin encountering social, psychological, or physical consequences.

As regular use continues, physiological adaptation of the body begins, and the individual's need for the drug in order to function normally increases. Without the drug, the person experiences the physical discomfort associated with withdrawal.

Until withdrawal is present, there may be little evidence that the user has progressed to the stage of *dependency*. Avoiding withdrawal is the motivational factor for people to continue to use. The individual not only needs drugs and/or alcohol to experience pleasure but, more importantly, to avoid physical and psychological distress on discontinuation of the drug.

But, as previously stated, physical dependence alone does not constitute an addiction. The defining conditions for addiction also include tolerance and, more importantly, psychological dependence. On average, it may take from 5 to 10 years following the first experimental use of drugs until a person progresses to the stage of dependency. Some individuals may be able to reverse this process, but this is rarely accomplished without outside help.

As use progresses through these stages, related physical, social, and psychological problems increase. Each stage entails some risk of progression to the next, but this course is not inevitable (Institute of Medicine, 1990b). Once the state of dependency is reached, the individual has acquired a chronic relapsing disorder. Return to earlier stages of controlled use is highly unlikely.

However, treatment is available to assist addicted individuals to enter a stage of *recovery* during which they abstain from use and experience improved physical, social, and psychological functioning. Because of *relapse*, the recovery process may be interrupted by periods of return to use. This requires attention to relapse prevention and continuing supportive therapeutic interventions.

SUMMARY

Why is it that many people use drugs for years without becoming addicted? Knowledge of the mechanisms of abuse and addiction has not advanced enough to provide a cogent understanding of the reasons some people manage their alcohol and/or drug use while others progress to addiction.

CHAPTER 3

ALCOHOL AND THE BRAIN

- **Basic Overview of Neuroscience**
- **Neurochemistry of Alcohol**

In addition to understanding terminology and key concepts, it is also important to have a basic understanding of neuroscience and the pharmacology of alcohol. This provides a foundation on which to build when managing the medical needs of patients. It also aids in understanding why patients exhibit certain physical, behavioral, cognitive, and other impairments as a result of traumatic injuries.

The use of alcohol by humans goes back thousands of years to the dawn of civilization. Today, the use of alcohol is a great problem in our society because it directly and indirectly affects everyone's lives. Concerned groups have raised their voices to stop alcohol abuse and its destruction of human life. The medical community has been given the job of investigating how alcohol affects different organs and the body as a whole.

Over the past three decades, there have been great changes in the nature of addiction in society, ranging from changing views of the nature of alcoholism, through the explosion of a drug culture in the 1960s, to the crack epidemic of the 1980s. In parallel, the potential for medical help for these problems has increased, beginning with the discovery in the early 1950s of pleasure or reward centers in certain brain regions, areas that we are now beginning to understand in terms of nerve pathways and neurochemistry.

Today, technology and education have aided scientists in penetrating the barriers of enigma that have halted the understanding of alcohol and its effects on the human brain.

BASIC OVERVIEW OF NEUROSCIENCE

The *nervous system* is composed of the *brain*, the *spinal cord*, and the *nerves*, which act together to serve as the communicating and coordinating system of the body. The system has two main divisions: the *central nervous system* (CNS) and the *peripheral nervous system* (PNS). The CNS comprises the brain and spinal cord. It integrates information and coordinates all bodily activities; the PNS is responsible for muscle coordination and impulses from sensory receptors throughout the body. The PNS is subdivided into the *somatic* and the *autonomic* nervous systems.

The Brain

The command center is the brain. It is contained within the *cranium*, and is connected at its base with the spinal cord (Tortora & Grabowski, 1993). It is protected from harmful substances in the blood stream by a barrier, referred to as the *blood-brain barrier*. This barrier keeps some substances out of the brain entirely and delays the entry of others.

The *cerebrum*, the main portion of the brain, is made up of an outer coating, or *cerebral cortex*, that controls many of the brain's functions; one of its important functions is complex cognition. Underneath the cerebral cortex are the *basal ganglia*, which are important in the maintenance of muscular tension. When these structures are exposed to certain psychoactive drugs, or are damaged by disease, it results in muscular rigidity in the arms, legs, and facial muscles.

The cerebral cortex covers the *cerebral hemispheres* which are connected by a pathway of nerve fibers called the *corpus callosum* (Figure 3–1). The two hemispheres are symmetrical and apparently identical, but they perform different functions. The left hemisphere is dominant for speech, analytical capabilities, and verbal and auditory memory in most people. The right hemisphere controls spatial and visual perception, creativity, and nonverbal memory (Tortora & Grabowski, 1993). When damage is sustained to the left hemisphere of the brain, language func-

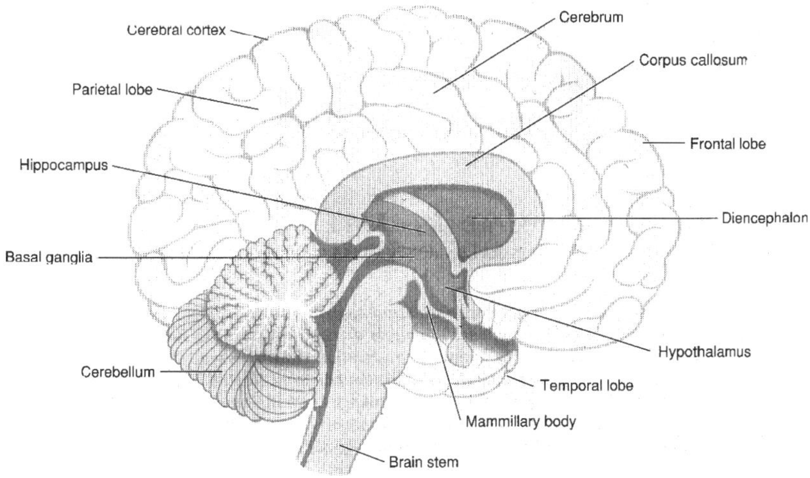

FIGURE 3–1. The brain's division of labor. (From *Alcohol Health & Research World, 19,* p. 137. Copyright 1995 by the National Institute on Alcohol Abuse and Alcoholism. Reprinted by permission.)

tions are often severely disrupted. When damage is sustained to the right hemisphere of the brain, subtle behavioral changes occur involving the individual's personality, emotional state, perception of the three-dimensional world, as well as changes in gross motor function (Oscar-Berman, 1992).

The Brain's Division of Labor

Each hemisphere is divided into four lobes, each with a highly specialized function (refer to Figure 3–1). The *frontal lobe* controls voluntary muscle movements, houses the motor area for speech, and controls emotional behavior and complex intellectual abilities. The *parietal lobe* receives and interprets sensory impulses from the skin, muscles, joints, and tendons. Sensations processed in this lobe include pain; heat; cold; pressure; recognition of the size, shape, and texture of objects; recognition of the location and intensity of various stimuli; and awareness of body parts. The *occipital lobe* receives and interprets visual stimuli, and the temporal lobe contains the centers for hearing, taste, and smell. The *temporal lobe* also receives and interprets sounds as words (Luckmann & Sorenson, 1974).

Beneath the cortex, within the cerebral hemispheres, lies the *thalamus*. The thalamus acts as a relay station for information related to sensation and movement. It is here that the *cordate nucleus* and *cerebellum* are found. They help to coordinate body movements and maintain balance.

The brain's lowest portion, called the *brain stem*, connects the cerebral hemispheres with the spinal cord. The brain stem regulates the basic physiological functions such as heart rate, respiration, eating, and sleeping, all of which can be affected by various drugs.

The *hypothalamus*, sometimes referred to as the body's emotional brain, is located at the base of the cerebrum. It participates in the regulation of metabolism, blood sugar levels, and body temperature, and directs activity and rest, appetite and digestion, sexual desire, and menstrual and reproductive cycles.

On top of the brain stem and below the cerebral cortex resides another set of structures called the *extrapyramidal areas* and the *limbic system*. The extrapyramidal area controls movement. The limbic system is a group of structures that are crucial in connecting the cortex with our emotions and motivations. These connections allow us to experience a wide range of feelings and to influence these feelings with our perceptions and actions. They also enable us to use our cognitive abilities to help us do the things we need to do to survive. Two major structures in the limbic system, the *hippocampus* and *amygdala*, are critical for short-term memory and learning (Figure 3–2) (NIAAA, 1994).

One of the reasons that psychoactive substances can exert such control over behavior is that they act directly on the brain stem and limbic structures, which can override the cortex in controlling our behavior. The *medial forebrain bundle* is often thought to be part of the limbic system. This collection of nerve fibers connects groups of cell bodies with areas of the limbic system that activate the *reward center*. It has been proposed that drugs that have the ability to act directly on the limbic system stimulate a "reward mechanism" that reinforces or leads to drug use. In essence, the reward center biologically reinforces any behavior that elicits a response of pleasure. The more the person learns to repeat the drug-taking behavior to produce pleasure, the more the brain learns to depend on the drugs to evoke pleasure. This is one of the key reasons why people repeatedly use drugs.

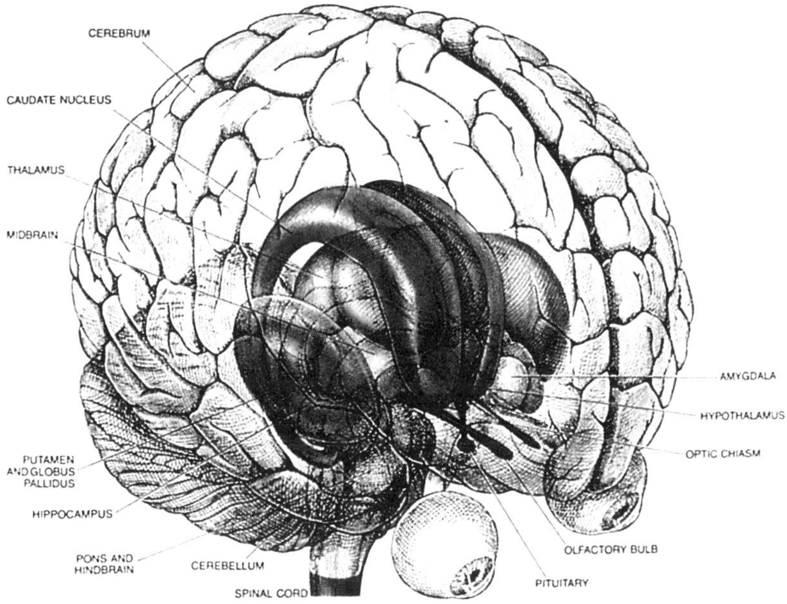

FIGURE 3–2. The human brain. (From "The Organization of the Brain," by W. J. H. Naua and M. Feirtag, 1979, *Scientific American, 241*, p. 102. Copyright 1979 by Scientific American, Inc. All rights reserved. Reprinted with permission.)

Neurons and Neurotransmission

The brain is comprised of billions of *neurons*—cells responsible for transmitting electrochemical impulses between one another. These electrochemical impulses take place by secretions of *neurotransmitters*—chemical messengers released by stimulated nerve cells.

At the head of the neuron is the *cell body*. Extending out from the cell body are fingerlike projections called *dendrites*. When a neuron is activated, an electrical impulse is generated at the cell body and passes along one long white-sheathed fiber called an *axon*, branching out and continuing into a network of *axon terminals*. This end of the nerve is referred to as the *presynaptic* nerve ending. Once the impulse reaches the presynaptic nerve ending, neurotransmitters are released from *synaptic vesicles*. These neurotransmitters then cross a small *synaptic gap* (or *cleft*), a tiny gap that separates the axon terminals of the transmitting neuron from the dendrites of the receiving or *postsynaptic* neuron (Figure 3–3).

Once the neurotransmitter is released the impulse is sent across the synaptic gap to bind to protein *receptors*, located in the outer membrane of the dendrites of the adjacent cell. Each receptor site is shaped so that it only binds to one specific neurotransmitter. This binding action is sometimes referred to as a *lock and key mechanism*. It is important to note that several different receptors may exist for each neurotransmitter (NIAAA, 1994). If the signals received by the postsynaptic neuron are strong enough, the neuron reaches an excitatory threshold and begins the process of information flow. The receptor molecules link with other molecules that extend through the cell membrane to the inside of the cell, consequently changing the cell's behavior. This change may consist of a transient increase or decrease in the neuron's responsiveness to further messages. Some receptors promote long-term changes that support functions such as growth, learning, or adaptation to changes in the neuron's environment, such as the presence of alcohol. The process of converting messages from other neurons into changes within the receiving neuron is called *signal transduction* (Shep-

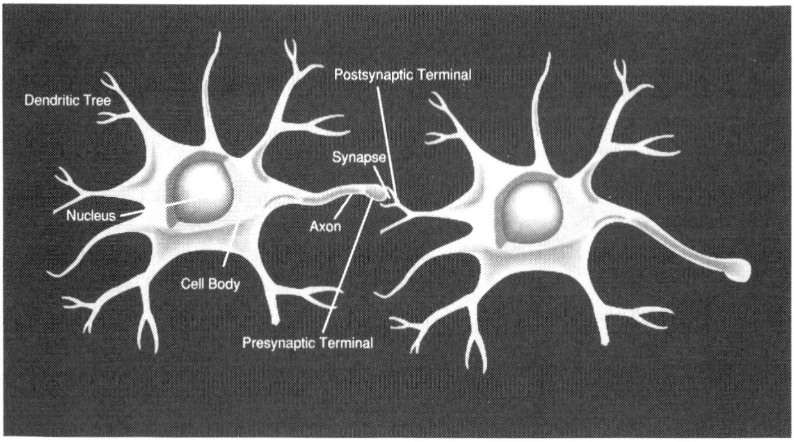

FIGURE 3–3. Cytology of two connected neurons. This schematic drawing illustrates the major components of neuronal structure including the dendrite tree, cell body, nucleus, axon, and synaptic connection. (From "Alcohol and the Brain," by M. Charness, 1990, *Alcohol Health & Research World, 14*, p. 87. Reprinted by permission.)

herd, 1994). Limited research suggests alcohol may produce some of its effects by interfering with signal transduction (Davis-Cox, Fletcher, Turner, Szarowski, & Shain, 1996).

Once the receptor activates these other molecules, its mission is complete. The reaction is terminated when the neurotransmitter is either reabsorbed by the nerve cell that released it or it dissipates. This process of electrical chemical communication is called *neurotransmission.* (Charness, 1990).

Any step in the communication process just described is a potential site of action for alcohol, tobacco, and other drugs. Some drugs may mimic or enhance the effects of the natural neurotransmitters at the receptor site (an *agonistic* action), or they may occupy the receptor site and prevent the neurotransmitter from activating it (an *antagonistic* action). Still others may interfere with the reabsorption of the neurotransmitter by the cell that released it (Ray & Ksir, 1993). When alcohol or drugs interfere with the normal activities of neurotransmission, they change the way the nerve cell functions and consequently have an impact on the way we feel and behave. It is also important to note that, unlike nearly all cells in the body, neurons cannot reproduce. If the brain's neurons divide, the intricate connections among the cells may be hopelessly disrupted; we are born with nearly our full complement of brain neurons, and those that die are lost forever (Swerslow, 1995; Tortora & Grabowski, 1993).

Neurotransmitters and Neurotransmission Pathways

As previously stated, several neurotransmitters exist. They fall into categories according to their effects on the postsynaptic neurons or according to their chemical structure. *Excitatory neurotransmitters* stimulate the cell to produce an electrical signal of its own, thus transmitting the signal to additional cells. *Inhibitory neurotransmitters* reduce the postsynaptic cell's sensitivity to signals, preventing further transmission. Some of the most important neurotransmitters with respect to alcohol are *norepinephrine*, *dopamine*, *acetylcholine*, *gamma-aminobutyric acid*, (GABA), and *serotonin* (also called 5-hydroxytryptamine or 5-HT) (Synder, 1987).

Acetylcholine. This neurotransmitter participates in the mechanism that is responsible in part for learning, memory formation and retrieval, conservation of energy, attention, defense or aggression, thirst, sexual behavior, mood, play, and rapid eye movements (REM) during sleep. Acetylcholine pathways arise from cell bodies in the basal ganglia and extend to the hippocampus and most of the cerebral cortex. Through these pathways, acetylcholine neurons respond to messages from the internal and external environment and deliver an integrated physiological and behavioral response (Ray & Ksir, 1993).

Dopamine. The essential action of dopamine is to relay nerve messages about pleasure from the brain stem to nerve cells in a limbic structure called the *nucleus accumbens.* This information is then relayed through another set of fibers to a related part of the frontal region of the cerebral cortex which is responsible for feeling pleasure. This is referred to as the *mesolimbic dopamine pathway.* Positron Emission Tomograpy (PET) scanning has shown that this pathway becomes highly active when impinged upon by all major drugs of abuse.

Dopamine fibers also arise in the *substantia nigra* in the midbrain and end in the basal ganglia. This pathway is referred to as the *nigrostriatal dopamine pathway.* It is this pathway that is damaged in Parkinson's disease and is affected by the tranquilizers that produce muscle rigidity as a side effect (Cohen, 1988; Ray & Ksir, 1993).

Serotonin. Serotonin-mediated pathways arise from the *raphe nuclei* and affect mood, sleep, the consumption of drugs, the development of tolerance to alcohol and other drugs, and the sensation of pain (Cohen, 1988; Ray & Ksir, 1993).

Norephinephrine. This neurotransmitter produces an alerting, attention focusing, orienting response. It dilates the pupils, increases heart rate and blood pressure, constricts most arteries, and decreases gastrointestinal activity. The pathways containing norepinephrine arise from the *locus ceruleus* and have numerous branches that project up and down the brain.

Gamma-aminobutyric Acid (GABA). This is an inhibitory neurotransmitter. It is not organized into discrete pathways or bundles and is found in most areas of the central nervous system. Alcohol and benzodiazepines interfere with the inhibitory effects of GABA, resulting in the potentiation of the effects of the drug (NIAAA, 1994).

NEUROCHEMISTRY OF ALCOHOL

The type of alcohol that human beings consume is called *ethanol*, which is the product of fermented fruits and grains.

Once alcohol has been absorbed, it enters the bloodstream to be metabolized and transported throughout the body. There are no brain receptors for alcohol as there are for other addictive drugs such as the opiates.

The mechanism of the depressant action of alcohol on the CNS is unknown; this is also true of all other generalized CNS depressants. Investigations of their primary mode of action have succeeded principally in characterizing secondary consequences of action. Individual neurons are less excitable, repolarize more slowly after excitation, and exhibit reduced spontaneous electrical activity. In addition, synaptic transmission is impaired.

The brain's long-lasting adaptations to alcohol may result in part from changes in gene function (Miles, 1995). Genes direct the synthesis of proteins, such as receptors. By influencing gene function, alcohol may alter the structure and function of specific receptors that have roles in intoxication, reinforcement, and physical dependence (Ortiz et al., 1995). Alcohol's effects on genes may also alter proteins involved in signal transduction (Davis-Cox et al., 1996).

Alcohol's effects on the neurotransmitters may contribute to the anxiolytic, sedative, and motor impairment actions of alcohol (Tabakoff, Hoffman, & Peterson, 1990). This is particularly true of the neurotransmitter GABA.

Serotonin is a neurotransmitter that is associated with the reinforcing effects of alcohol, consequently leading to continued use. Research has shown that alcoholics tend to have low serotonin levels. Thus, it is believed that consuming alcohol increases the levels of serotonin. This suggests the possibility that alcohol intoxication may be an attempt to self-medicate low serotonin levels (Tabakoff et al., 1990). This also explains the experimental use of serotonin uptake inhibitors and other serotonergic drugs to reduce heavy alcohol consumption. Drugs that inhibit serotonin uptake by neurons prolong the action of serotonin by allowing it to persist in the synapse (Tabakoff et al., 1990).

Alcohol consumption also increases norepinephrine (NE), resulting in altered sleep patterns and changes in temperature regulation during and after withdrawal (Tabakoff et al., 1990). NE release and activity increases at the time of alcohol withdrawal especially during the period when symptoms are most evident, but NE remains elevated after many of the acute symptoms of alcohol withdrawal disappear.

In addition, alcohol produces an increase in the levels of dopamine in the nucleus accumbens, and also increases dopamine metabolism in other brain areas thought to be involved in the brain reinforcement system. However, when tolerance develops, the neurotransmitter's production is not so readily increased by alcohol (Tabakoff et al., 1990). There is evidence that decreased activity in neurons using this neurotransmitter may play a significant role in the presence and severity of certain withdrawal symptoms (e.g., depression) (Tabakoff et al., 1990).

GABA, the major inhibitory neurotransmitter in the CNS, is part of a larger protein complex that includes a channel for the passage of chloride ions into the cell. When GABA interacts with the receptor, chloride entry into the neuron is increased, rendering the neuron less sensitive to the effects of other neurotransmitters (Tabakoff et al., 1990). There is now substantial evidence that tolerance to alcohol's sedative effects may be the result of an adaptation of the GABA-controlled ion channels to the chronic presence of alcohol.

Although GABA is the major inhibitory neurotransmitter in the CNS, the amino acid glutamate is the major excitatory neurotransmitter in the brain. There are several subtypes of glutamate receptors. Alcohol affects primarily one known as the N-methyl-D-asparate (NMDA) receptor. This receptor is believed to play a role in learning and memory, neuronal development, seizures, and brain damage resulting from a lack of oxygen (Tabakoff et al., 1990). Activation of the NMDA receptor by glutamate results in a large uptake of calcium by the neuron, which increases the responsiveness of the neuron to stimuli. This increased sensitivity could contribute to CNS hyperexcitability during alcohol withdrawal. This hyperexcitability in turn may contribute to such withdrawal symptoms as anxiety, tremors, increased heart rate, and seizures (Tabakoff et al., 1990).

Calcium may also enter the neuron secondary to changes in the neuronal membrane. In acute consumption, alcohol temporarily inhibits or reduces calcium uptake, thus reducing transmitter release and depressing neuronal communication. Whereas, in long-term use, alcohol leads to an increase in a group of calcium channels called *L-channels* (Tabakoff et al., 1990). As a result, the action potential is affected, as well as the individual's self-control, by slower reactions to stimuli.

Depending on amount, the effects of alcohol on the brain include excitation, intoxication, and uncoordination, and a sedative effect similar to that of depressants. At higher doses, alcohol leads to unconsciousness; and at very high doses, its depressant effects on the respiratory center can be fatal. Alcohol has a profound effect on the frontal lobe—the part of the brain that allows us to analyze and program our behavior. These processes require a tremendous amount of energy; the depressant nature of alcohol directly lowers the energy center in the brain and, as a result, mental capacity is lost (Tabakoff et al., 1990).

SUMMARY

Neuroscience research has led to a better understanding of the effects of long- and short-term alcohol consumption on brain function. In addition, research has provided insight into the mechanisms by which alcohol produces its intoxicating and behavioral effects. "Heavy alcohol consumption causes impairments in the way that information is transmitted in the brain. Alcohol induces changes in nerve cells and chemical messengers that influence the development of intoxication, tolerance, and the symptoms of withdrawal" (Tabakoff et al., 1990, p. 138).

CHAPTER 4

ALCOHOLISM, ALCOHOL USE, AND ABUSE

- Definition of Alcoholism
- Tolerance and Dependence
- Understanding Disabilities and Alcohol Abuse

According to a recent article by Joseph Beasley (1995), "there are 18 million alcoholics in this country and almost 1 in 5 Americans (18%) lives with an alcoholic while growing up" (p. 2). The consequences of alcohol abuse on society are staggering. Totaling both direct costs for treatment and medical care for alcohol-related illnesses and injuries and indirect costs associated with crime and violence, property loss, and loss of productivity, the annual cost may be as high as $120 billion (Moos, Finney, & Cronkite, 1990).

The medical as well as the lay community has struggled with defining the problem for decades. Various views worth mentioning have included moral failing, medical disease, mental disorder, behavioral condition, and a culturally induced form of social deviance. The contemporary stand today is that alcoholism is a treatable entity. Alcoholism, like mental illness, is in no way related to social or economic class. It is equally common among the rich and the poor, the intelligent and the mentally limited, the successful and the unsuccessful.

Aside from caffeine, alcohol is used by more people, and in larger quantities, than any other psychoactive substance. Alcoholic beverages have been consumed by humans since the dawn of time (Neolithic man drank berry wine in 6400 B.C.), and efforts to regulate consumption have gone on for centuries (Ray, 1983).

According to the National Institute on Alcohol Abuse and Alcoholism, 7% of adult Americans (an estimated 13,760,000) abused or were dependent on alcohol during 1992. In 1995, the prevalence of alcohol abuse and dependence was highest among respondents aged 18–24, regardless of sex or ethnicity (Center for Substance Abuse Treatment [CSAT], 1995). Over 30% of teenagers aged 14–17 have used alcohol and other drugs and paid the consequences: arrests, highway crashes, crime, violence, arrests for driving while intoxicated (DWIs), health problems, impaired school and job performance, and death.

Today, alcohol remains the most commonly abused substance among adolescents—given the early onset of drinking and its frequency, the consequences of alcohol's acute and chronic effects on physiological growth and maturation, as well as its potential effects on the development of social and interpersonal competencies, are of a major concern.

Alcohol abuse contributes to four leading causes of death in men before the age of 45: cirrhosis, suicide, homicide, and automobile accidents. It also increases the risk of stroke, dementia, compromises the myocardium and the immune system, and may accelerate physical deterioration. Alcohol-related problems increase the incidence of stressful life events, impair mental health, and compromise social supports (Vaillant, Schnurr, Caron, & Gerber, 1991).

DEFINITION OF ALCOHOLISM

In 1956, the American Medical Association labeled alcoholism a "disease." This classification followed many years of slowly shifting public attitudes and opinions. The American Psychiatric Association followed suit in 1965 and the American Bar Association and the American Medical Association issued a joint declaration in support of the disease concept in 1969 (Kinney & Leaton, 1991).

To provide a basis for discussion, this book will use the definition of alcoholism provided by the National Council on Alcoholism and Drug Dependence (NCADD) and the American Society of Addiction Medicine (ASAM):

> A primary chronic disease with genetic, psychosomatic, and environmental factors implicated in its development and manifestations. The disease often progresses and is fatal. It is characterized by continuous or periodic impaired control, overdrinking, preoccupation with the drug alcohol, use of alcohol despite adverse consequences, and distortions in thinking, most notably denial. (Morse & Flavin, 1992 p. 1012)

NCADD and ASAM further say that by "discase" they mean "involuntary disability," and that the symptoms of alcoholism may be continuous or may occur periodically. Further, the two groups say that the development of alcoholism in a person is influenced by genetic, psychosocial, and environmental factors, and that the disease of alcoholism is often progressive and fatal.

Social stigma has blocked the road to the understanding of alcoholism more than with any other disease. Society has long viewed the affliction as a psychological problem alone—the sign of a ravaged soul devoid of discipline or morality. Health care professionals tend to ignore its symptoms and its victims deny its existence.

Recent scientific breakthroughs, however, have begun to dramatically alter our views on alcoholism. The myth that alcoholism is a "psychological problem" is yielding under the weight of evidence that the disease has its roots in biological causes. Such discoveries may eventually lead to prevention or detection of the disease before its damage becomes irreversible.

TOLERANCE AND DEPENDENCE

Tolerance and dependence may promote increased alcohol consumption. As you may recall, tolerance means that after continued drinking, consumption of a constant amount of alcohol produces a lesser effect or increasing amounts of alcohol are necessary to produce the same effect. The development of tolerance allows and encourages increased intake of alcohol because more of the drug is required to achieve the same effects.

Tolerance to alcohol also results in cross-tolerance, decreasing the effectiveness of other sedatives such as benzodiazepines and barbiturates. Therefore, alcoholics undergoing withdrawal may require very large doses of benzodiazepines to produce sedation. It is important to note that tolerance to different effects of alcohol develops differentially, varying in extent, persistence, and perhaps even in the neurological mechanisms involved.

Individuals who are becoming alcohol dependent begin to experience a loss of control. They may hide their drinking (e.g., sneak drinks or wear heavy perfume), gulp the first drink, participate in "predrinking" drinking, experience gaps in memory, and be unwilling to discuss their drinking. Embarrassing episodes cause shame, guilt, decreasing self-esteem, trouble in close relationships, verbal and physical abuse, and perhaps dangerous accidents. Individuals develop anxiety, fear, and guilt when drinking because they never know when they will lose control (Brown, 1994).

They may also begin to lose their health and sense of basic safety. They may minimize the amount of alcohol consumed; rationalize their use of alcohol (used as medicine or because of problems); change their drinking pattern; organize activities around drinking; display marked self-pity; neglect appearance; neglect eating; protect their supply; become aggressive at times, even abusive; lose interest in other activities; and become a danger to themselves and to others, a terrifying fact that must be denied. The individuals begin to drink continuously or in prolonged binges. They become confused and their thinking is impaired. They experience tremors and will drink alcohol products (e.g., vanilla extract, mouthwash) to relieve the signs of withdrawal. The pathology of active alcoholism is centered on the denial of loss of control, the very reality that is the source of repeated, inescapable trauma (Brown, 1994).

Characteristics of Alcoholism

Characteristics of alcoholism that contribute to the devastating impact of the disease include:

- Alcoholism is a progressive disease that generally first appears between ages of 20 and 40, although children can become alcoholics.
- Drinking patterns vary by age and sex. At all ages, two to five times more males than females are heavy drinkers. For both males and females, drinking prevalence is highest and abstention lowest in the

21 to 34 age range. Among those 65 years and older, abstainers exceed drinkers in both sexes.

- Alcohol dependence tends to cluster in families.
- Alcohol dependence is often associated with depression. Depression typically makes its appearance before the drinking. Studies show that, among the general population, those with diagnosable depression are at a somewhat elevated risk for development of alcoholism. Among women, however, the risk is tripled.
- Women seem also to be more sensitive to alcohol than men. When differences in weight are factored out women still seem to get higher blood levels of alcohol from drinking—a fact that may increase their risk.
- It takes 5 to 15 years for an adult to become an alcoholic; an adolescent can become an alcoholic, by contrast, in 6 to 18 months of heavy drinking. Younger alcohol abusers are also more likely to die of alcohol poisoning through hypoglycemia because their livers cannot metabolize the alcohol as effectively as the adult liver. Alcohol overdose itself may also be fatal.
- Generally, abuse occurs in one of three patterns: regular, daily intoxication; drinking large amounts of alcohol at specific times, such as a weekend; and long periods of sobriety interspersed with binges of heavy daily drinking that last for weeks or months.
- As drinking continues, dependence develops and sobriety brings serious withdrawal symptoms such as delirium tremens (DTs), which includes physical trembling, delusions, hallucinations, sweating, and hypertension.
- Long-term, heavy drinking can cause dementia, in which the individual loses memory and the ability to think abstractly, to recall names of common objects, to use correct words to describe recognized objects, or to follow simple instructions.
- Physical complications of chronic alcohol dependence include cirrhosis, hepatitis altered brain-cell functioning, nerve damage, gastritis, premature aging, impotence and infertility, and a variety of reproductive disorders. It also increases the risk and severity of heart disease, pneumonia, tuberculosis, and neurological disorders.

In contrast to physical dependence is psychological dependence, characterized by craving for the drug. Psychological functioning becomes distorted by the development of a massive defensive barricade. Denial (the outright rejection of the realities of drinking), magical thinking, minimization, grandiosity, and omnipotence are all utilized to help the individual manage the feelings and other consequences produced by these experiences. The individual begins to lose and destroy everything that has been important. Consequently, individuals may often feel terrified, helpless, and out of control (Bean-Bayog, 1986).

UNDERSTANDING DISABILITIES AND ALCOHOL ABUSE

The passage of the Americans with Disabilities Act (ADA) of 1990 was a significant landmark for people with disabilities. The increased public awareness stemming from the ADA has focused attention on a variety of disability issues that previously were ignored. One such issue is the relationship between disabilities and the risk for alcohol problems. As societal myths about disabilities disappear, people with disabilities can acknowledge that they are subject to the same dilemmas experienced by others.

A Definition of Disability

The ADA (1990) defines a person with a disability as anyone who either:

- has a physical and/or mental impairment that substantially limits one or more major life activities; or,
- has a record of such an impairment; or,
- is regarded by others as having such an impairment. (Department of Justice, p,469)

The increased level of awareness on alcohol abuse and disabilities is timely. The burdens that alcohol pose are compounded when the individual is one of the estimated 43 million Americans who have one or more physical or mental disabilities. For these individuals, the process of recovery is made more difficult by barriers that do not exist for others.

According to the Resource Center on Substance Abuse Prevention and Disability, alcohol is significantly more prevalent among people with disabilities. People with disabilities often use medication over extended periods of time, with multiple prescriptions. The medications may influence behavior or interact with other drugs, such as alcohol. The special medical conditions associated with some disabilities can decrease alcohol tolerance. There may be a corresponding increase in risk for accidents due to preexisting balance, mobility, or visual impairments. People who experience chronic pain are more likely to either become dependent on prescribed medications or use other drugs, such as alcohol, to attempt temporary release from the discomfort. Alcohol problems that existed prior to the disability tend to continue and worsen.

With the onset of a disability, a family may experience additional expenses, difficult adjustments to daily routines, and reduced income due to loss of job. Such factors significantly increase stresses that can lead to unhealthy behaviors. The negative reactions to a disability can include shock, denial, anger, depression, resentment, guilt, and embarrassment. Family, friends, and professionals may inadvertently encourage people with disabilities to misuse alcohol (Kraus, 1992). Enabling may be motivated by misplaced feelings of compassion, guilt, frustration, or camaraderie. (Enabling describes attitudes and behaviors of others that give the individual with an alcohol problem either direct or indirect permission to continue alcohol abuse and dependence.)

People with disabilities may have fewer opportunities for association with peer groups. Societal prejudice and social limitations can result in gravitation to peer groups that tolerate or encourage alcohol use. Lack of transportation or recreational or social opportunities frequently isolates persons with disabilities from others. This can lead to depression, poor self-esteem, and alcohol misuse. When a person has limited social options, it can be difficult to change friends in order to avoid negative influences. Underemployment or unemployment, financial concerns, and lack of access to alcohol treatment resources and services also contribute to the overall prevalence of alcohol abuse.

SUMMARY

The United States has always had a serious alcohol problem; peak per capita consumption occurred in the 1820s or earlier. Approximately 43 million Americans meet the ADA disability criteria. Although the nature of their disabilities varies, all share an increased risk for alcohol abuse. Clearly, people with disabilities may abuse alcohol for all the same reasons as their nondisabled peers. However, the higher risk reflects a direct relationship to the existence of a disability.

CHAPTER 5

CONSEQUENCES OF ALCOHOL USE AND ABUSE

- Biochemical Effects of Alcohol Metabolism
- Adverse Consequences of Alcohol Consumption
- Nutritional Deficiencies Related to Alcohol Consumption

Heavy and chronic drinking can harm virtually every organ and system in the body. In this chapter, information about the biochemical effects of alcohol metabolism and its effects on body systems is presented.

BIOCHEMICAL EFFECTS OF ALCOHOL METABOLISM

Alcohol is quickly and efficiently absorbed from the gastrointestinal tract into the circulatory system and transported to the liver for metabolism; it also may be metabolized in the stomach (NI-

AAA, 1994). The rate of absorption depends on the concentration of alcohol, the amount and type of food in the stomach, and whether or not the liquid is carbonated. Diluted alcohol is absorbed more slowly than a highly concentrated "shot" of liquor. However, if the diluent is carbonated or the alcoholic product itself is effervescent, it will pass more rapidly into the small bowel and be absorbed even faster than in the stomach. Eating foods containing fat and/or protein before or while drinking alcohol delays absorption (Porth, 1994; Shlafer, 1993).

The Role of THIQ in Alcoholism

When a normal individual drinks alcohol, it is metabolized at a rate of approximately 10 ml per hour (but is quite variable with weight, age, gender, etc.). The alcohol is converted to acetaldehyde, which is very toxic, and the body quickly converts this to acetic acid. The acetic acid is then converted into carbon dioxide and water, which are eliminated through the kidneys and lungs. This same process occurs in the alcoholic, but with an additional twist. In the alcoholic, a small amount of the acetaldehyde is not metabolized into acetic acid. Instead, it goes to the brain and interacts with dopamine to become tetrahydroisoquinoline (THIQ). THIQ is never excreted. It accumulates, in small amounts, in the brain each time the individual consumes alcohol. THIQ is highly addictive (Ohims, 1990). Potential alcoholics have inherited a predisposition toward the production of THIQ in their brain chemistry. This predisposition is usually not known to them. As a result, potential alcoholics may begin as moderate social drinkers, but each time alcohol is consumed, a small amount of THIQ is formed and stored in the brain. Again, production of THIQ occurs only in the brains of alcoholics, it does not occur in the brains of normal social drinkers. At some point, the levels of THIQ cross a threshold; this threshold is the dividing line between social drinking and addiction (Ohims, 1990).

Effects are noticed approximately 10 minutes after consumption and peak at approximately 40–60 minutes. In order to be excreted, alcohol is changed in the liver by the enzyme *alcohol dehydrogenase* (Lieber, 1976). Because alcohol cannot be stored in the body and very little can be excreted by the lungs or kidneys, it will remain in the bloodstream unchanged until metabolized by the liver. The blood-brain barrier allows the remaining alcohol to pass readily from the circulating blood into the brain cells (Cataldo, Debruyne, & Whitney, 1992; Porth, 1994), consequently affecting neurotransmission.

In addition, excessive alcohol intake may lead to the formation of ethanol-fatty compounds known as *fatty acid ethyl esters.* It is hypothesized that these compounds may compromise protein synthesis and reduce the amount of energy produced by the cell.

The average adult can metabolize approximately 10 ml of ethyl alcohol per hour, which is somewhat less than the amount of alcohol in one 12 ounce beer (4%–5% alcohol) or a 4-ounce glass of wine (10%–12% alcohol). If an individual consumes alcohol at a faster rate than it can be metabolized, the blood alcohol level will rise (Shlafer, 1993). The initial metabolic product is acetaldehyde, a compound that may play a central role in alcohol toxicity (Shlafer, 1993).

Cocaethylene: The Dangerous Combination of Cocaine and Alcohol

When cocaine is combined with alcohol consumption, users are compounding the danger each drug poses and unknowingly forming a complex chemical experiment within their bodies. In 1991, researchers at the University of Miami School of Medicine found that the human liver combines cocaine and alcohol and manufactures a third substance, cocaethylene (Ray & Ksir, 1993; Schuckit, 1989). Cocaethylene increases both the euphoria and the craving associated with cocaine, while potentially increasing the risk of sudden death.

Acute ethyl alcohol ingestion inhibits the liver's drug metabolizing enzyme systems; chronic ingestion stimulates them. Both effects contribute to important drug interactions. Enzyme stimulation by chronic ingestion of ethyl alcohol also contributes to the development of tolerance and cross-tolerance (Shlafer, 1993). Some of this tolerance can be explained by the induction of enzymes in the liver, which allows faster metabolism, and some by brain tolerance, an adaptation to the neuropsychological effects of alcohol.

Physical dependence develops after years of heavy consumption, after which abstinence results in delirium tremens, leading to possible seizures and death.

ADVERSE CONSEQUENCES OF ALCOHOL CONSUMPTION

As recently discussed, alcohol is rapidly absorbed through the stomach and passes readily through the blood-brain barrier. The most widely held theory of alcohol action is through direct effects on the membranes of nerve cells.

Alcohol supplies a large caloric yield (7 cal/gram) without supplying any nutrition, and damage to the gastrointestinal (GI) tract further impairs absorption of vitamins. Many of the effects of alcohol on the CNS are attributed to a combination of direct alcohol damage and vitamin deficiencies (Table 5–1) (Cataldo et al., 1992).

Neurological Disorders Related to Alcohol Consumption

Multiple neurologic effects are associated with acute or chronic alcohol exposure. Alcohol has immediate effects on an individual's mental and motor abilities. These include slurred speech, drowsiness, irritability, behavioral changes, loss of restraint, loss of inhibition, loss of coordination, and a combination of exhilaration and excitement (Arria, Tarter, & Van Thiel, 1990). The next sections discuss the acute and chronic effects of alcohol abuse.

Acute Neurologic Effects of Alcohol

Mild symptoms of acute alcohol intoxication, such as altered mood, impaired cognition, and uncoordination develop at low blood alcohol concentrations (BACs) (.025%). These symptoms have been attributed to neurochemical disruptions in neuronal pathways (previously described in Chapter 3) in the brain stem, cerebral cortex, and cerebellum (Klemm, 1979). At higher BACs (0.1%) additional signs appear, such as involuntary rapid eye movements, double vision, speech disorders, and lack of muscular coordination. Involvement of the autonomic nervous system may result in hypotension, hypothermia, stupor, coma (Lehman, Pilich, & Andrews, 1993), and possible death if BACs higher than 0.5% are attained (Charness, Simon, & Greenberg, 1989).

Table 5–1. Alcohol related disorders.

Problem	*May Be Experienced*	*Causes*
Esophagitis	Vomiting, nausea, pain in the front or back of neck, any point behind the breast bone. The pain can be burning in nature, can be in spasms, can be aggravated by solid food or hot liquids or acidic fluids like coffee or alcohol. Blood might be vomited. It is usually bright red if not from stomach.	1. Direct effects of concentrated alcoholic beverages. 2. Irritable nervous system along with local irritation can cause spasms or retching and vomiting that can tear lining and walls of the gullet. 3. Enlarged blood vessels due to local effects, liver trouble and retching can cause breakdown of lining—this is ulceration. 4. Nutritional status.
Esophageal carcinoma	Pain is usually quite clear; definite point pain is experienced along the course of the gullet. Swallowing of fluids and food may be impaired. The food may be blocked at a definite point.	1. Prolonged local irritation due to excessive alcohol use. 2. Heavy smoking. 3. Black males have high incidence. 4. Exact steps to cancer from irritation are not fully known, but the relationship is well established.
Gastritis	Burning pain, nausea, vomiting, acidic taste of vomited material. Blood may be present.	1. Direct effect of concentrated alcohol beverages and prolonged contact with alcohol. 2. Irritable nervous system. 3. Increased acid production due to irritated nervous system, alcohol effect, chemicals that have accumulated because liver is not functioning well, and smoking. 4. Nutritional status. 5. Irritating beverages.
Malabsorption	Vitamins are not absorbed, causing: *Neuritis (B1)* 1. Feelings of pins and needles in glove and stocking areas. 2. Loss of pain and tempertature sensation. Touch is preserved, but burning oneself can occur.	1. Alcohol intake can replace food intake as a source of calories. 2. Alcoholic vomiting, etc., due to gastritis can reduce intake, digestion, and absorption. 3. Liver injury can impair digestion and absorption of fats, vitamins A, D, E, K.

continued

Table 5–1. *continued*

Problem	May Be Experienced	Causes
	3. Wasting of muscles. *Brain Damage (B1, B3)* Confusion, cross-eye gaze, and bizarre behavior. ❖ Heart can be weakened with poor circulation. Severe dry patchy skin (B3). ❖ Severe diarrhea (B3). ❖ Problem with anemia (B12). ❖ Spinal cord damage (B12). Increased risk of infections. Clotting of blood can be slow (Vitamin K deficiency). Aging of body tissues increased. Liver function impaired due to protein deficiency.	4. Pancreas failure impairs digestion of proteins, fats. 5. Presence of alcohol in small intestine blocks vitamins B12, B1, B3, amino acid absorption. 6. Chronic diarrhea reduces absorption.
Chronic diarrhea	Repeated liquid bowel movement; weakness.	Problems with digestive function of stomach, liver, pancreas, small bowel due to alcohol.
Pancreatitis	Severe pain in the back and lower abdomen; vomiting; poor digestion; hypotension; fever; tachycardia; blood sugar fluctuations; diaphoresis.	Heavy alcohol abuse causing: ❖ blockage of emptying tube from pancreas; ❖ problems with fat increasing production of pancreatic juice; ❖ increased acid production by stomach due to alcohol increases production of pancreatic juice; and ❖ infection due to stagnant juices worsens problem.
Cirrhosis	Nausea, anorexia, weight loss. Abdomen and lower extremities may be swollen. Black stool or bloody vomit.	1. Alcohol abuse over a 10–15 year span. 2. Fatty liver and hepatitis can lead to cirrhosis. 3. By-products of alcohol metabolism. 4. Associated drug abuse (heroin, barbiturates).

Problem	*May Be Experienced*	*Causes*
Cardiomyopathy	Edema of lower extremities. Difficulty breathing. Reduced urine formation.	1. Direct effect of alcohol on heart. 2. Change in the fatty substances in circulatory system due to alcohol.
Beriberi	❖ If heart involved, similar to cardiomyopathy. ❖ If nerves involved, similar to peripheral neuritis. Dry Beriberi is called Wet Beriberi when the heart is involved.	1. B1 deficiency impairing the chemical reactions of the heart. 2. B1 deficiency can be caused by alcohol use in spite of adequate nutrition.
Duodenal ulcer	Pain after ingestion of food in upper portion of stomach. Dark vomit. Poor nutrition. Narrowing and blockage with severe vomiting. Severe hemorrhage.	1. Psychological stress, anger, frustration, severe tension. May be alcohol related. 2. Vulnerability of duodenum (hereditary). 3. Increased acid production due to alcohol consumed; failure of damaged liver to destroy acid producing chemicals.
Fatty liver	Poor digestion, nausea, heavy sensation in right side. Fatty liver changes to become hepatitis if alcohol abuse continues.	1. Direct effect of alcohol oxidation on liver cells: toxic by-products encourage deposition of fat. 2. Poor diet with too many calories and fat can worsen condition.
Alcoholic hepatitis	Potentially lethal. Fever, enlarged liver, jaundice, increased white blood count, clay stools, dark stools, dark urine. Liver test can prove it is due to alcohol. Symptoms mistaken for gallstones. Hepatitis can go to cirrhosis or liver failure if drinking continues.	1. Direct effect of alcohol abuse. Heavy prolonged or heavy sudden drinking in person without tolerance. 2. Other infections (viral) and drugs can worsen condition.
Peripheral neuropathy	Pins and needles-like sensations. Pain and temperature sense dulled or	1. Malabsorption of vitamin B1 due to blocking effect of alcohol on absorption of

continued

Table 5–1. *continued*

Problem	***May Be Experienced***	***Causes***
	lost. Small injuries may become worse. Wasting of muscles supporting wrist, ankle, concerned with movement.	nutrients in bowel. 2. Poor nutrient intake (both quantitatively and qualitatively), vomiting and diarrhea (due to poor appetite and gastriocolitis). 3. Vitamin B1 deficiency can lead to death of nerves.
Convulsions	Loss of consciousness, may be mild or severe. Stiffening of all muscles with a board-like or bow-shaped form. Repeated jerky movement, affecting trunk, neck, eyes, upper and lower extremities. In some cases an odd sensation—visual or mental—precedes convulsion. Symptoms vary among individuals.	1. Unknown cause. 2. Due to viruses; rabies. 3. Due to infection of nervous system; meningitis, encephalitis, tetanus. 4. Due to vitamin B6 deficiency when antibiotic drugs are used. 5. Due to scars or blood clots in the brain from injuries (80–90% of brain blood clots are among alcoholics). 6. Increased irritability of the brain and nerves when a person is coming off a period of drinking. Maximum risk from 48–72 hours. 7. Low blood sugar.
Alcoholic hallucinosis	Commonly people hear voices. These voices may evoke violent behavior toward self, others, or property.	1. May be underlying emotional disturbance brought on by drinking. 2. May occur due to loss of coordination and control within an irritable nervous system as the individual experiences alcohol withdrawal.
Delirium tremens	Changing levels of awareness. Individual at one time is completely alert and at another is disoriented. Confusion, severe shakes, agitation, anxiety, hallucinations may occur, high fever and/or infection may be present. Death occurs in 10–15% of untreated cases.	1. Alcohol or sedative (e.g., barbiturates) withdrawal is reason for DTs. The type of drug use that precedes is more important than quantity or period. 2. High level of alkaline substances in blood influence both the confused state of the brain and the severe shakes.

Problem	*May Be Experienced*	*Causes*
Wernicke's syndrome	Individual consuming alcohol develops confusion, changed level of consciousness, symptoms of neuritis.	Directly related to vitamin B1 deficiency. (Refer to , malabsorption and peripheral neuritis.)
Korsakoff's psychosis	Recent memories may be lost. Old memories remain clear. May create stories to cover memory loss. Confusion with regard to person, place, time, etc.	Vitamin B1 deficiency, malabsorption syndrome, blood clotting.
Marchiafava's syndrome	Severe mental malfunction. Because behavioral symptoms are not specific, diagnosis is rarely made except at autopsy.	Combination of nutritional deficiency and effects of alcohol on blood supply to the brain.
Myopathy	Periodic cramping, swelling, weakness; in chronic cases, muscles may be destroyed with weakness.	Chronic alcohol abuse affects muscles directly through mechanisms not completely understood. Seems to be independent of nutritional status, but related to effects of alcohol on enzymes of muscles.
Anemia	Weakness, dizziness, breathlessness with exertion, may be associated with decreased pain and temperature sensation. Muscles of lower extremities can become spastic.	1. Vitamin B12 and folic acid due to poor intake and malabsorption. 2. Destruction of stomach lining which excretes chemical required to absorb B12.
Pellagra	Dry scaly, dark pigmented patchy skin on exposed parts of body, especially legs. Diarrhea, dementia, confusion, poor memory.	
Scurvy	Gums become ulcerated and teeth may fall out. Cuts do not heal.	Vitamin C deficiency.
Hypoglycemia	Irritability, seizures, tremulousness, diaphoresis, fainting spells, muscle weakness, headache, hostility, impulsivity, suicidal feelings.	Liver disease; insulin-producing tumor in pancreas; metabolic abnormalities involving brain, adrenal glands, and possibly pituitary glands.

continued

Table 5–1. *continued*

Problem	*May Be Experienced*	*Causes*
Hyperglycemia	Increased respirations, fruity odor to breath, cold palms, faintness, tachycardia, weakness.	1. Diabetes mellitus. 2. Stimulation of adrenal glands from alcohol.

Pathological Intoxication

As previously mentioned, alcohol is a depressant with effects that extend to the brain and spinal cord. However, for a small percentage of individuals, alcohol excites rather than sedates. Individuals affected by this disorder will exhibit aggressiveness and assaultive and destructive behavior, even after consuming only a small quantity of alcohol. These individuals will have outbursts of rage and destructive behavior toward others, with no recall of the incident when sober. This is called a *pathological intoxication* (Lehman et al., 1993).

Alcoholic *blackouts*—transient episodes of amnesia that cannot be attributed to loss of consciousness, seizures, head trauma or *Wernicke-Korsakoff syndrome* (WKS)—also result from consumption of large quantities of alcohol. During a blackout, the individual appears conscious but has no recall of the event when sober. These blackouts are caused by alcohol's ability to suppress neuronal activity in the brain and to slow the transmission of signals within the brain (Lehman et al., 1993). All of these acute symptoms may affect individuals with or without alcoholism.

Alcohol Withdrawal Syndrome

Alcohol-dependent individuals who cease drinking or reduce their alcohol intake undergo a withdrawal process that may vary in severity. Withdrawal can be separated into three distinct clinical syndromes. The most common is mild in nature, occurs within 24 to 36 hours after cessation of drinking, and is characterized by restlessness, anxiety, sleeping problems, agitation, and tremor. Tachycardia, low-grade fever, or diaphoresis may also develop, as well as an elevated blood pressure (Fleming &

Barry, 1992). The second stage is characterized by signs and symptoms of the first stage, plus visual and auditory hallucinations; signs and symptoms may begin as soon as 24 hours after the last drink or be delayed for up to 72 hours. Alcoholic hallucinosis is distinguished from delirium tremens by the fact that the patient is not markedly agitated, is not disoriented, and realizes that the experience is unreal (Fleming & Barry, 1992). Patients may become increasingly agitated and frightened. Tremors may involve the whole body, heart rate is greater than 100, and diaphoresis becomes more pronounced. Vomiting may occur (Fleming & Barry, 1992; Porth, 1994).

The final stage is the development of delirium tremens (DTs). The delirium in alcohol withdrawal commonly manifests itself by disorientation, global confusion, and an inability to recognize familiar objects or persons. The clinical signs and symptoms are usually severe and the patient may or may not have hallucinations (Fleming & Barry, 1992; Naranjo & Sellers, 1986). Symptoms have been reported as early as 24 to 48 hours after cessation of drinking; however, it can take as long as 3 weeks to develop in some patients (Fleming & Barry, 1992).

Symptoms of Alcohol Withdrawal

Withdrawal symptoms may include:

- Restlessness
- Tachycardia
- Irritability
- Hypertension
- Anorexia
- Insomnia
- Nausea
- Nightmares
- Vomiting
- Impaired concentration
- Diaphoresis
- Impaired memory
- Tremor
- Elevated vital signs

More severe symptoms of alcohol withdrawal may include:

- Increased tremulousness
- Increased agitation
- Increased diaphoresis
- Delirium (with confusion, disorientation, impaired memory, and judgment)
- Hallucinations (auditory, visual, or tactile)
- Delusions (usually paranoid)
- Grand mal seizures

continued

continued

Note: Withdrawal symptoms do not necessarily progress from mild to severe. In some individuals, a grand mal seizure may be the first sign of withdrawal. Seizures usually occur 12 to 24 hours after cessation or reduction of drinking. One third of all patients who have seizures develop delirium tremens. Withdrawal seizures typically are grand mal, last less than 5 minutes, and are singular (Fleming & Barry, 1992).

As a final note, if a patient experiences a seizure during alcohol withdrawal, it does not automatically follow that the seizure is from alcohol withdrawal. Alcohol withdrawal seizures are rarely life-threatening unless they occur when the patient is in a hazardous environmental position (e.g., driving an automobile). In contrast, the underlying disease process of many other etiologies of seizures in this patient population are indeed life-threatening. Alcoholics have a high incidence of head trauma, so subdural hematoma as an etiology of seizures should be considered. Alcoholics are also at higher risk of infections, therefore, infectious etiologies of seizures should also be considered.

It is also important to address that phenytoin (Dilantin®) has not been shown to prevent alcohol withdrawal seizures. When started in a patient not previously on phenytoin, oral administration is not likely to reach a therapeutic blood level during the period of time the patient is most at risk for seizures. Even if a therapeutic blood level could be reached, there is no evidence that phenytoin is helpful in preventing alcohol withdrawal seizures (Alldredge, Lowenstein, & Simon, 1989).

Once the crisis of withdrawal is over, a wide variety of illnesses can surface. It is important to remember that alcohol withdrawal may not be the only crisis you and your patient will face. Today's alcoholics are increasingly likely to be abusing many drugs.

Brain Damage and Premature Aging

Chronic alcohol abuse accelerates the aging of the individual's brain by causing premature shrinkage of the brain tissue. Research has shown that the brain of an alcoholic is aged far beyond the individual's chronological age (Lehman et al., 1993; Oscar-Berman, 1992). Symptoms of atrophy are slurred speech, loss of limb coordination, swaying, and lack of balance. Many of these symptoms can be partially reversed by abstaining from alcohol and supplementing the diet with vitamins (Oscar-Berman, 1990).

Chronic Effects of Alcohol

Three categories of organic brain disease associated with chronic alcoholism have been distinguished in the recent literature, based on neuropsychological profiles: the Wernicke-Korsakoff syndrome, alcoholic dementia, and "nonamnesic" or non-Korsakoff disorders. The basic distinction among these groups is the presence or absence of amnesia and the severity of intellectual decline.

The best known of these syndromes is Wernicke-Korsakoff syndrome (WKS). WKS is caused by a deficiency of the B1 vitamin, thiamine, and really consists of two disorders. The first disorder is a motor disorder called *Wernicke's encephalopathy* and is characterized by mental disturbances such as extreme confusion, apathy, drowsiness, loss of coordination while walking, and constant nystagmus. When patients are treated with thiamine, their neurologic symptoms generally improve (Langlais, 1995; Victor, Adams, & Collins, 1989). Partial recovery may occur over 12 months; however, patients who recover from Wernicke's encephalopathy are sometimes left with a residential memory impairment called *Korsakoff syndrome*, the second disorder. Its most characteristic symptoms are anterograde amnesia, retrograde amnesia, and impairment of several cognitive processes (Jernigan & Ostergaard, 1995; Langlais, 1995; Oscar-Berman, 1990; Porsjesz & Begleiter, 1995).

The brains of individuals afflicted with this two-part disease have been found to have lesions in various areas. These lesions can vary from mild to severe, with total loss of brain tissue in the affected area. WKS is treated with abstinence from alcohol and thiamine supplements. Recovery can be partial or complete, depending on the severity of damage prior to treatment (DeSoto, O'Donnell, & DeSoto, 1989; Lehman et al., 1993; Oscar-Berman, 1992; Porth, 1994).

Alcoholic dementia is distinguished from WKS by global intellectual deterioration in addition to severe memory impairment (Cutting, 1978; Lishman, 1986). In addition, dementia patients have relatively intact intellectual abilities (Butters & Cermak, 1980), gradual rather than acute onset of symptoms, and a longer drinking history. Patients tend to show improvement with abstinence.

The third neuropsychologically defined group, non-Korsakoff disorders, show no overt behavioral signs of profound cognitive dysfunction. Deficits are subtle in nature and typically include impairments in abstraction ability and problem solving, impairments in visuoperceptual abilities, and mild learning and memory deficits. As in the other two groups, there is significant recovery following abstinence (Ryan & Butters, 1986).

In addition to the previously described neurological disorders, alcohol is a contributory factor in the development of polyneuropathy and amblyopia. With regard to polyneuropathy, the distal portions of the legs are the first and most severely affected. Pain and numbness may develop. However, this is not true in all cases. For some, these symptoms may be absent, and the diagnosis may be made on the basis of muscular wastage, calf tenderness, impaired motor and sensory innervation, and reduced knee and ankle jerks (Hofmann, 1983). Progression of this disorder may occur over time, involving the upper extremities. Partial recovery may require years, and permanent disabilities frequently occur.

Amblyopia is a bilateral and symmetrical loss of visual acuity for both near and far objects. As with polyneuropathy, this disorder is believed to result from a nutritional deficiency. Optic nerve degeneration may occur if treatment is inadequate (Hofmann, 1983).

Additional Physiological Consequences of Alcohol Consumption

The Gastrointestinal Tract

Alcohol metabolism affects many other biochemical pathways of the body. Starting at the top of the gastrointestinal system, the oral cavity suffers from neglect leading to dental caries, lesions of the lips, gums, and tongue, periodontal disease, hypersensitivity, and impaired healing. In the esophagus there is pyloric valve relaxation and reflux, erosion, and esophageal varices. The stomach, which absorbs 20% of the alcohol, may develop ulcerations and symptoms of gastritis. The effects of alcohol on the intestines, where the remaining 80% of the alcohol is absorbed, are numerous and include duodenal-gastric reflux/ulcer, enzyme inhibition, diminished integrity/repletion, diarrhea, and hyper- and hypomotility.

The Pancreas

The effects of alcohol on the pancreas have long been recognized. Impairment of pancreatic function and liver glucose synthesis may cause life-threatening hypoglycemia or coma. Acute pancreatitis is characterized by destruction of the acinar cells' membrane (acinar cells secrete enzymes necessary for digestion) and inflammatory damage to blood vessels (Singh, 1990). Chronic relapsing pancreatitis is more commonly associated with alcoholism than acute pancreatitis (Korsten, 1989).

The Liver

Chronic alcohol abuse is unquestionably the single most important cause of liver disease in the United States. Alcohol-induced liver disease progresses from fatty liver to chemical or alcoholic hepatitis, with jaundice, fever, elevated white cells, and a 30% mortality rate. Alcoholic (chemical) hepatitis is a bridge between fatty liver and hepatic hepatitis. All blood flows from the GI tract through the liver; cirrhosis may cause hypertension in these pathways, with gastrointestinal (GI) varices (veins) and bleeding, which may be fatal. Abdominal ascites or hepatic delirium or coma may occur. Seventy-five percent of all cases of pancreatitis stem from alcohol ingestion, presenting with severe pain, elevated serum amylase readings, and, in extreme cases, diabetes (Grant, Dufour, & Harford, 1988; Korsten, 1989).

The Stages of Alcoholic Liver Disease

The liver is the primary site for alcohol metabolism. Consequently, the liver is highly susceptible to alcohol-induced injury. Alcoholic liver disease usually progresses in three distinct stages. The first stage is the development of a fatty liver, which is a reversible condition that is accompanied by only slight tissue damage. At this stage, little evidence of liver dysfunction is detected. The second stage is alcoholic hepatitis and fibrosis. These two disorders represent a more

continued

continued

serious condition than fatty liver. They are associated with increasing destruction of liver tissue and consequently with increasing liver dysfunction. Alcoholic hepatitis results in inflammation and destruction of the liver tissue. In alcoholic fibrosis, healthy liver tissue is replaced by scar tissue. The final stage of alcohol-induced liver disease is alcoholic cirrhosis. A cirrhotic liver is characterized by heavily scarred liver tissue and a lumpy (nodular) appearance. Coinciding is severe dysfunction, which in turn can impair the functioning of other organs and contribute to disorders such as kidney failure, gastrointestinal bleeding, lowered resistance to infections, ascites, esophageal varices, poor blood clotting, folic acid deficiency anemia, hepatic coma, and brain disorders (NIAAA, 1994).

Fatty liver is reversible with abstinence, alcoholic hepatitis is usually reversible upon abstinence, and although alcoholic cirrhosis is often progressive and fatal, it can stabilize with abstinence (Rubin, 1989).

The Cardiovascular System

Other complications of alcoholism range from congestive heart failure, hypertension (Friedman, 1990; Lands & Zakhari, 1990), and cardiac arrhythmias, to cardiomyopathy and stroke (Zakhari, 1991). In excessive amounts, alcohol causes coronary artery disease, secondary to atherosclerotic narrowing (narrowing caused by plaque formation) (Klatsky, 1990), and increases the workload of the heart (Friedman, 1992; Rubin & Doria, 1990; Urbano-Marquez et al., 1989). The association of sudden cardiac arrthymias with alcohol abuse, generally without evidence of heart disease, has been given the phrase *holiday heart* (Messerli, 1993).

Alcohol also decreases the bone marrow's ability to make red blood cells, causing anemia; it reduces the number of white blood cells and destroys platelets, causing a person to bruise easily by interfering with normal blood clotting. Alcohol also causes swelling of the arteries in the head that puts pressure on nerves, resulting in headaches, and it widens veins near the surface of the skin, resulting in loss of body heat.

The Endocrine System

The endocrine system releases chemical mediators called hormones into the circulation to act on other remote tissues. At the level of the hypothalamus and pituitary, there is a link between the nervous and endocrine systems that integrates the two systems into one functional unit. Hormones are involved in such diversified domains as reproduction; growth and development; maintenance of body fluids, electrolytes, and temperature; and regulation of blood pressure and heart rate, to name a few. Alcohol affects not only the synthesis and release of hormones, but also their transport interaction with tissues and metabolism (NIAAA, 1994).

Numerous studies have clearly demonstrated the adverse effects of alcohol abuse on gonadal function. These include inflammation of the prostate gland causing inhibited sexual function, testicular atrophy (Lloyd & Williams, 1948), lowered testosterone levels, lowered sperm counts, diminished sexual drive, impotence, and gynecomastia.

With respect to females of child-bearing age, chronic alcohol abuse has been associated with menstrual cycle irregularities such as amenorrhea (complete cessation of menses) and anovulaton (failure to ovulate). Alcoholic women were also found to have a higher rate of early menopause (Gavaler, 1988) and higher frequencey of menstrual irregularities (duration, flow, or both) than nonalcoholic women (Becker, Tonnesen, Kaas-Claesson, & Gluud, 1989).

Fetal Alcohol Syndrome

Alcohol use during pregnancy can seriously harm a developing fetus and affects women from all social and economic groups (Finnegan & Kandall, 1992). It is estimated that 1 to 3 in 1,000 babies born each year in the United States are born with significant prenatal alcohol exposure. These numbers increase to 10 in 1,000 among some Native American groups. Fetal Alcohol Syndrome (FAS) and Fetal Alcohol Effects (FAE) are the most notable adverse effects of alcohol exposure during pregnancy. Alcohol is the leading preventable cause of mental retardation.

During the embryonic stage of development (from the second through the eighth week after conception), the fetus is particularly vulnerable to the effects of alcohol. This is the period crucial to the development of the brain and vital organs, and during which the central nervous system is differentiated from the other organ sys-

continued

continued

tems. Yet it is also a time when a woman might not know she is pregnant and so might not temper her alcohol use. Thus, it is essential that a woman be counseled about the dangers of perinatal alcohol use before she becomes pregnant. It is not known what level of alcohol consumption during pregnancy may be considered safe, so health care professionals are most often counseled to recommend that women who are pregnant or trying to conceive, abstain from alcohol use.

FAS is characterized by a cluster of congenital birth defects that develop in the infants of some women who drink heavily during pregnancy. These defects include pre- and postnatal growth deficiency; skull or brain malformations, such as microencephaly (abnormal smallness of the head), a flattened midface, sunken nasal bridge, and flattened and elongated philtrum; central nervous system dysfunction; and varying degrees of major organ malformation.

Although recent evidence indicates that the number of women who consume alcohol during pregnancy is declining, it appears that the rates of alcohol consumption among high-risk populations (pregnant smokers, unmarried women, women under the age of 25, and women with the least amount of education) remain unchanged (Serdula, Williamson, Kendrick, Anda, & Byers, 1991). This emphasizes the need to develop better targeted prevention and education efforts to reach high-risk populations and to identify women at high risk through primary health care and other systems.

The Immune System

Chronic alcohol abuse depresses the immune system and results in a predisposition to infectious disease (Garro, Espina, & Lieber, 1992; Lieber, Garro, Leo, & Worner, 1986), consequently leading to a variety of illnesses (Gluckman, Dvorak, & MacGregor, 1977; Mutchnick & Lee, 1988; Nelson, Shellito, Mason, & Summer, 1992; Roselle, 1992) including an increased susceptibility to bacterial infections, tuberculosis (Jacobson, 1992), and cancer (MacGregor, 1986; Mufti, Darban, & Watson, 1989). This effect of alcohol may be significant in immunocompromised patients, such as those with HIV infection. Before exposure to alcohol weakens the body's immunity to the AIDS virus, and after infection has occurred, alcohol may influence the activation of HIV (Bagasra, Kajdacsy-Balla, & Lischner, 1989). As infection progresses into the development of AIDS-related symptoms, alcohol contributes to the ability of a secondary infection to overcome the immune system (Kruger & Jerrells, 1992; Nair et al., 1990).

Other important actions of alcohol include depression of the release of antidiuretic hormone creating a build-up in uric acid crystals, leading to the development of kidney stones, gout, and swelling in the joints. It irritates, sedates, and kills tissue cells; reduces the ability to smell and taste; dehydrates tissue, causing halitosis and dental problems; and depletes calcium, resulting in weak bones and muscles (Bjorneboe et al., 1988; Hingson & Howland, 1987; Rico, 1990).

Alcohol also stimulates the production of some steroid hormones that in turn stimulate the adrenal glands to secrete, hormones that affect metabolism. The most dramatic result of this hormone excess is pseudo-Cushing's syndrome.

NUTRITIONAL DEFICIENCIES RELATED TO ALCOHOL CONSUMPTION

The nutritional effects of alcohol abuse are of more than just academic interest. Admission to hospitals for malnutrition related to alcoholism remains significant. Alcoholism is suggested as the most common cause of vitamin and trace-element deficiency in adults in the United States (Miller & Gold, 1991).

Chronic heavy drinking is associated with deficiencies in many vitamins because of decreased food ingestion and, in some cases, impaired absorption, metabolism, and utilization (Lieber, 1988, 1989). For example, alcohol inhibits fat absorption and thereby impairs absorption of the vitamins A, E, and D, which are normally absorbed along with dietary fats (Leo & Lieber, 1989; Lieber, 1989). Vitamins A, C, D, E, K, and B, also deficient in some alcoholics, are all involved in wound healing and cell maintenance (Tortora & Anagnostakos, 1987). In particular, because vitamin K is necessary for blood clotting, deficiencies of that vitamin can cause delayed clotting and result in excess bleeding.

Even when food intake is adequate, alcohol can impair the mechanisms by which the body controls blood glucose levels, resulting in either increased or decreased blood glucose (Patel, 1989). As a result, alcohol causes the brain and other body tissue to be deprived of glucose needed for energy and function.

Nutritional deficiencies resulting from dietary insufficiency from concomitant liver disease can compound the effects of alcohol on the brain. Vitamin B deficiencies are common in alcoholic patients. Thiamine (vitamin B1) is necessary for normal energy metabolism, appetite, nervous system function, and the synthesis of new cells. Alcohol-induced liver injury impairs the activity of the liver enzyme that activates thiamine. Chronic B1 deficiency can precipitate Wernicke's encephalopathy. Other vitamin B deficiencies are associated with neurologic disturbance (e.g., peripheral neuropathies and ocular motor palsies).

Folate is necessary for the synthesis of new cells (especially blood cells and GI cells). In the presence of alcohol, the body excretes folate from all sites of action and storage. Thus, alcohol abuse causes a folate deficiency that devastates the digestive system and impairs the oxygen-carrying capacity of the blood.

Vitamin A deficiency is a primary cause of nightblindness (McClain, Van Thiel, Parker, Badzin, & Gilbert, 1979) and vitamin E deficiency is associated with a neurologic syndrome characterized by ataxia, neuromuscular weakness, and motor incoordination (Feinman, 1989; Sokol, Iannaccone, Bove, & Heubi, 1983).

SUMMARY

The consequences of alcohol abuse affect almost every part of the body. An understanding of the physiological consequences of alcohol abuse is necessary to adequately identify and assess patients in a hospital setting. It is important to remember that alcoholism may not be part of the admitting diagnosis, but when it exists it will complicate other conditions.

CHAPTER 6

SCREENING AND ASSESSMENT FOR ALCOHOL DEPENDENCY IN THE HOSPITALIZED PATIENT

- **Screening Questionnaires and Interviews**
- **Assessing for Alcohol Use and Abuse**

In the general hospital, health-related professionals are in a prime position to identify the alcohol-dependent patient. Too often, though, professionals miss this opportunity for early identification. The most meaningful indicators of alcohol abuse are more often than not difficult to assess. Psychological and behavioral signs usually become evident before the development of physical disorders. Physical findings cannot be relied on as they are often late manifestations (Glaze & Coggan, 1987).

Clues That May Assist in Identification of an Alcohol Problem

- A patient's failure to respond to standard doses of tranquilizers or sedative. A regular drinker who has developed tolerance is not going to sleep after one sleeping capsule.
- Mood swings. A patient may grow agitated and tremulous before visiting hours, then become calm, even euphoric, afterward.
- Overabundance of mouthwash or toiletries. (One patient on a surgical unit developed DTs after 2 weeks in the hospital; the source of his alcohol was after-shave lotion.)
- Physical signs of chronic alcohol use, such as tremors or periorbital and pretibial edema caused by fluid retention after a drinking bout.
- Frequent references to alcohol or alcohol use, indicating the importance of alcohol in the individual's life.
- Physical signs of current drinking, such as alcohol on breath, flushed face caused by vasodilitative effects of alcohol.
- Multiple bruises, burns, or abrasions at different stages of healing. These appear most frequently at table-top height or on the hands and face and are caused by falls and accidents when intoxicated.
- Slash marks on wrists from suicide attempts associated with the depression of chronic alcoholism.
- An older appearance than stated age. The debilitating effects of prolonged, excessive use of alcohol can result in premature signs of aging.

The patient who is obviously intoxicated when admitted to the hospital is not necessarily an alcoholic; however, staff should be alert to the possibility. Unless medical staff documents alcohol signs of intoxication when the patient is admitted, one to two shifts later, the staff on the unit may be puzzled and totally unprepared when patient becomes anxious and disruptive for no apparent reason. Keep in mind that even a nonalcoholic who has a regular drinking pattern can experience the agitation of mild withdrawal when the pattern is disrupted by hospitalization. For the alcohol-dependent patient who has suffered a trauma or who has a preexisting disability, the staff's failure to assess alcohol use can be catastrophic.

SCREENING QUESTIONNAIRES AND INTERVIEWS

Alcohol is primarily or secondarily implicated in a large number of medical problems. Screening for alcohol use is a critical component of hospital management of the patient with traumatic injuries. In addition, screening is the basis for identifying persons at risk for reinjury because of underlying alcohol problems.

It is important to remember that laboratory tests alone are not adequate to screen for alcohol dependency; they simply detect the presence or absence of alcohol in body fluids and thus indicate recent use. Effective screening depends on interpretation of these results in the context of other information about frequency and pattern of alcohol and other drug use.

Patterns of Alcohol Use

Studies have shown that one-third or more of patients with traumatic injuries who test positive for alcohol have at least one other drug in their system (Clark & Harchelroad, 1991). The presence of alcohol should be a red flag for the presence of other drugs.

The issue of polydrug use provides further reason for screening of trauma patients. As previously discussed, several organ systems can be involved in a single traumatic injury. That fact, coupled with the high incidence of polydrug use, compounds the complexity of treating the patient. The information gained from screening can be an important aid in assessing injury and how it should be treated.

Brief information about several available screening and assessment instruments that may be utilized in a hospital setting are described here. An additional list is included in the Appendix. The instruments included in this book do not represent an exhaustive exploration of all such instruments, nor does incorporation in this list represent an endorsement of particular instruments. Rather, these are offered as a compilation of instruments located through literature review.

Alcohol Screening Questions

Very often, patients present in a hospital setting because they are in need of medical intervention. When interacting with the patient, it is important to remember that the alcoholic may be in a state of denial or ambivalence about the need for treatment (Senay, 1992).

If the patient reports drinking, questions pertaining to drinking history should be asked. These generally include onset of drinking and age of first intoxication, years of problematic drinking, drinking locations and contexts, reasons for drinking, family history of drinking problems, drinking patterns, and quantity and frequency of alcohol intake. Gently elicit the truth through open and easy questions. Try not to push the patient or engage in confrontation. Several questions have been recommended. Examples of questions include: "How many days per week to do you drink?" (frequency); "On a day when you drink, how many drinks do you have?" (quantity); and "How many times in the last month did you drink more than five drinks at one sitting?" (binge drinking) (Rostenberg, 1995).

There are, however, both limitations and variations in the accuracy of patient responses to such questions. Patients may underestimate alcohol consumption because of denial or forgetfulness. Others may wish to conceal the information for fear of the associated social stigma (Dean & Poremba, 1983) or punitive action by employers and law-enforcement officials. To minimize problems of inaccurate self-reporting, it is important to ask about specific amounts of drinking; to define a single drink; to inquire about specific amounts of beer, wine, and hard liquor; and to inquire about the frequency, quantity, and occasions of heavier use with separate questions (Cutler, Wallace, & Haines, 1988).

Inquiries also need to be made about history of hangovers, shakes, seizures or convulsions, loss of control drinking, hallucinations, delirium tremens, memory impairment and blackouts, tolerance, and drinking to alleviate withdrawal symptoms. Finally, questions regarding earlier attempts to resolve drinking problems, such as making efforts to reduce drinking without help of formal treatment, attending meetings of Alcoholics Anonymous (AA), or participating in previous treatment programs should be asked (Maisto & Connors, 1990).

Alcohol Screening Tests

Michigan Alcoholism Screening Test (MAST)

The MAST (Selzer, 1971) (Figure 6–1), is a self-report 25-item questionnaire that focuses on the consequences of problem drinking and on the subjects' perception of their alcohol problems (Mattox, 1986). It is important to note that the MAST is the only screening instrument that has been extensively validated for use with trauma patients.

CAGE

The CAGE questionnaire is a self-report screening instrument that indicates alcohol-related problems (Allen, Eckardt, & Wallen, 1988; Ewing, 1984; Ewing & Rouse, 1970), poses four overt yes-no questions, and requires approximately 1 minute to complete. The score is the number of "yes" answers (0 to 4). A score of two positive answers strongly suggests alcoholism (Mayfield, McLeod, & Hall, 1974). It may be useful as part of the routine medical screening process. It asks the following four questions:

- C: Have you ever felt you should *Cut down* on drinking?
- A: Have people *Annoyed* you by criticizing your drinking?
- G: Have you ever felt bad or *Guilty* about your drinking?
- E: Have you ever had a drink first thing in the morning to steady your nerves or get rid of a hangover *(Eye-opener)*?[1]

Alcohol Use Disorders Identification Test (AUDIT)

The AUDIT can be used to accurately diagnose early as well as severe alcohol problems and includes information about quantity and frequency of alcohol use past and present (Isaacson, Butler, Zacharedk, & Tzelepis, 1994; Saunders, Aasland, Babor, De La Fuente, & Grant, 1993).

[1]From "Detecting Alcoholism: The CAGE Questionnaire," by J. A. Ewing, 1984, *Journal of the American Medical Association, 252*, p. 1907. Copyright 1984 by the American Medical Association. Reprinted with permission.

MICHIGAN ALCOHOLISM SCREENING TEST (MAST)

YES NO Points

*0. Do you enjoy a drink now and then?
____ ____ (1)

*1. Do you feel you are a normal drinker?
(By normal we mean you drink less than or as much as most other people.)
____ ____ (2)

2. Have you ever awakened the morning after some drinking the night before and found that you could not remember a part of the evening?
____ ____ (2)

3. Does your wife, husband, a parent, or other near relatives ever worry or complain about your drinking?
____ ____ (1)

*4. Can you stop drinking without a struggle after one or two drinks?
____ ____ (2)

5. Do you ever feel guilty about your drinking?
____ ____ (1)

*6. Do friends or relatives think you are a normal drinker?
____ ____ (2)

*7. Are you able to stop drinking when you want to?
____ ____ (2)

8. Have you ever attended a meeting of Alcoholics Anonymous (AA)?
____ ____ (5)

9. Have you gotten into physical fights when drinking?
____ ____ (1)

10. Has your drinking ever created problems between you and your wife, husband, a parent, or other relative?
____ ____ (2)

11. Has your wife, husband (or other family members) ever gone to anyone for help about your drinking?
____ ____ (2)

12. Have you ever lost friends because of your drinking?
____ ____ (2)

13. Have you ever gotten into trouble at work or school because of your drinking?
____ ____ (2)

14. Have you ever lost a job because of drinking?
____ ____ (2)

15. Have you ever neglected your obligations, your family, or your work for two or more days in a row because you were drinking?
____ ____ (2)

16. Do you drink before noon fairly often?

____ ____ (1)

17. Have you ever been told you have liver trouble? Cirrhosis?

____ ____ (2)

**18. After heavy drinking have you ever had delirium tremens (DTs) or severe shaking, or heard voices, or seen things that really weren't there?

____ ____ (2)

19. Have you ever gone to anyone for help about your drinking?

____ ____ (5)

20. Have you ever been in a hospital because of drinking?

____ ____ (5)

21. Have you ever been a patient in a psychiatric hospital or on a psychiatric ward of a general hospital where drinking was part of the problem that resulted in hospitalization?

____ ____ (2)

22. Have you ever been seen at a psychiatric or mental health clinic or gone to any doctor, social worker, or clergyman for help with any emotional problem, where drinking was part of the problem?

____ ____ (2)

***23. Have you ever been arrested for drunk driving, driving while intoxicated, or driving under the influence of alcoholic beverages?

____ ____ (2)

(IF YES, How many times? ________)

***24. Have you ever been arrested, or taken into custody, even for a few hours, because of other drunk behavior?

____ ____ (2)

(IF YES, How many times? ________)

* Alcoholic response is negative

** 5 points for delirium tremens

*** points for **each** arrest

SCORING SYSTEM: In general, five points or more would place the subject in an "alcoholic" category. Four points would be suggestive of alcoholism, three points or less would indicate the subject was not alcoholic.

Programs using the above scoring system find it sensitive at the five point level and it tends to find more people alcoholic than anticipated. However, it is a screening test and should be sensitive at its lower levels.

FIGURE 6–1. Michigan Alcoholism Screening Test (MAST). (From "The Michigan Alcoholism Screening Test: The Quest for a New Diagnostic Instrument," by M. L. Selzer, 1971, *American Journal of Psychiatry, 127*, p. 1655. Copyright 1971 by the American Psychological Association. Reprinted by permission.)

Particular strengths of the AUDIT in regard to screening of trauma patients are that it is designed for use in a primary health care setting, it provides early detection of hazardous and harmful drinking, and it focuses on present rather than lifetime use (Bohn, Babor, & Kranzler, 1995).

Simple Screening Instrument for Alcohol and Other Drug Abuse (SSI)

The SSI is a 16-item questionnaire (Figures 6–2 and 6–3) that also includes a clinical observation checklist for signs and symptoms of alcohol and other drugs of abuse.

Interview Form

Note: **Boldfaced questions** constitute a short version of the screening instrument that can be administered in situations that are not conducive to administering the entire test. Such situations may occur because of time limitations or other conditions.

Introductory statement:
"I'm going to ask you a few questions about your alcohol and other drugs during the past 6 months. Your answers will be kept private. Based on your answers to these questions, we may advise you to get a more complete assessment. This would be voluntary—it would be your choice whether to have an additional assessment or not."

During the past 6 months . . .

1. **Have you used alcohol or other drugs? (Such as wine, beer, hard liquor, pot, coke, heroin, or other opiates, uppers, downers, hallucinogens, or inhalants)** (yes/no)
2. **Have you felt that you use too much alcohol or other drugs?** (yes/no)
3. **Have you tried to cut down or quit drinking or using drugs?** (yes/no)
4. Have you gone to anyone for help because of your drinking or drug use? (Such as Alcoholics Anonymous, Narcotics Anonymous, Cocaine Anonymous, counselors, or a treatment program)
5. Have you had any of the following?
   - ❖ Blackouts or other periods of memory loss
   - ❖ Injury to your head after drinking or using drugs

- ❖ Convulsions, or delirium tremens ("DTs")
- ❖ Hepatitis or other liver problems
- ❖ Feeling sick, shaky, or depressed when you stopped drinking or using drugs
- ❖ Feeling "coke bugs," or a crawling feeling under the skin, after you stopped using drugs
- ❖ Injury after drinking or using drugs
- ❖ Using needles to shoot drugs

6. Has drinking or other drug use caused problems between you and your family or friends? (yes/no)
7. Has your drinking or other drug use caused problems at school or at work? (yes/no)
8. Have you been arrested or had other legal problems? (Such as bouncing bad checks, driving while intoxicated, theft, or drug possession) (yes/no)
9. Have you lost your temper or gotten into arguments or fights while drinking or using drugs? (yes/no)
10. Are you needing to drink or use drugs more and more to get the effect you want? (yes/no)
11. Do you spend a lot of time thinking about or trying to get alcohol or other drugs? (yes/no)
12. When drinking or using drugs, are you more likely to do something you wouldn't normally do, such as break rules, break the law, sell things that are important to you, or have unprotected sex with someone? (yes/no)
13. Do you feel bad or guilty about your drinking or drug use? (yes/no)

Now I have some questions that are not limited to the past 6 months.

14. Have you ever had a drinking or drug problem? (yes/no)
15. Have any of your family members ever had drinking or drug problem? (yes/no)
16. **Do you feel that you have a drinking or drug problem now?** (yes/no)

- ❖ Thanks for answering these questions.
- ❖ Do you have any questions for me?
- ❖ Is there something I can do to help you?

Notes:____

____

____

____

(continued)

(continued)

Observation Checklist

The following signs and symptoms may indicate an AOD abuse problem in the individual being screened:

- Needle track marks
- Skin abscesses, cigarette burns, or nicotine stains
- Tremors (shaking and twitching of hands and eyelids)
- Unclear speech: slurred, incoherent, or too rapid
- Unsteady gait: staggering, off balance
- Dilated (enlarged) or constricted (pinpoint) pupils
- Scratching
- Swollen hands or feet
- Smell of alcohol or marijuana on breath
- Drug paraphernalia such as pipes, paper, needles, or roach clips
- "Nodding out" (dozing or falling asleep)
- Agitation
- Inability to focus
- Burns on the inside of the lips (from freebasing cocaine)

FIGURE 6–2. Simple Screening Instrument for AOD Abuse. (From Simple Screening Instruments for *Outreach for Alcohol and Other Drug Abuse and Infectious Diseases* (Treatment Improvement Protocol (TIP) Series 11, DHHS Publication No. SMA 94-2094, pp. 12–13), by K. C. Winters and J. M. Zenilman, 1994, Rockville, MD: U.S. Department of Health and Human Services.)

Self-Administered Form

Directions: The questions that follow are about your use of alcohol and other drugs. Your answers will be kept private. Mark the response that best fits for you. Answer the questions in terms of your experiences in the past 6 months.

During the past 6 months . . .

1. Have you used alcohol or other drugs? (Such as wine, beer, hard liquor, pot, coke, heroin, or other opiates, uppers, downers, hallucinogens, or inhalants)
   _____ Yes   _____ No

2. Have you felt that you use too much alcohol or other drugs?
   _____ Yes   _____ No

3. Have you tried to cut down or quit drinking or using drugs?
   _____ Yes   _____ No

4. Have you gone to anyone for help because of your drinking or drug use? (Such as Alcoholics Anonymous, Narcotics Anonymous, Cocaine Anonymous, counselors, or a treatment program)
   _____ Yes _____ No

5. Have you had any of the following?

   - Blackouts or other periods of memory loss
   - Injury to your head after drinking or using drugs
   - Convulsions, or delirium tremens ("DTs")
   - Hepatitis or other liver problems
   - Feeling sick, shaky, or depressed when you stopped drinking or using drugs
   - Feeling "coke bugs," or a crawling feeling under the skin, after you stopped using drugs
   - Injury after drinking or using drugs
   - Using needles to shoot drugs

6. Has drinking or other drug use caused problems between you and your family or friends?
   _____ Yes _____ No

7. Has your drinking or other drug use caused problems at school or at work?
   _____ Yes _____ No

8. Have you been arrested or had other legal problems? (Such as bouncing bad checks, driving while intoxicated, theft, or drug possession)
   _____ Yes _____ No

9. Have you lost your temper or gotten into arguments or fights while drinking or using drugs?
   _____ Yes _____ No

10. Are you needing to drink or use drugs more and more to get the effect you want?
    _____ Yes _____ No

11. Do you spend a lot of time thinking about or trying to get alcohol or other drugs?
    _____ Yes _____ No

12. When drinking or using drugs, are you more likely to do something you wouldn't normally do, such as break rules, break the law, sell things that are important to you, or have unprotected sex with someone?
    _____ Yes _____ No

13. Do you feel bad or guilty about your drinking or drug use?
    _____ Yes _____ No

The next questions are about your lifetime experiences.

14. Have you ever had a drinking or other drug problem?
    _____ Yes _____ No

15. Have any of your family members ever had a drinking or drug problem?
    _____ Yes _____ No

(continued)

(continued)

16. Do you feel that you have a drinking or drug problem now?
_____ Yes _____ No

Thanks for filling out this questionnaire.

Scoring for the AOD Screening Instrument

Name/ID No.: ______________________ Date: __________________

Place/Location: ____

Items 1 and 15 are not scored. The following items are scored as 1 (yes) or 0 (no):

___ 2	___ 7	___ 12
___ 3	___ 8	___ 13
___ 4	___ 9	___ 14
___ 5	___ 10	___ 16
___ 6	___ 11	

Total score: ___ Score range: 0–14

Preliminary interpretation of responses:

Score	Degree of Risk for AOD Abuse
0–1	None to low
2–3	Minimal
≥4	Moderate to high: possible need for further assessment

FIGURE 6–3. Simple Screening Instrument for AOD Abuse. (From *Simple Screening Instruments for Outreach for Alcohol and Other Drug Abuse and Infectious Diseases* (Treatment Improvement Protocol (TIP) Series 11, DHHS Publication No. SMA 94-2094, p. 5), by K. C. Winters and J. M. Zenilman, 1994, Rockville, MD: U.S. Department of Health and Human Services.)

ASSESSING FOR ALCOHOL USE AND ABUSE

Early assessment is important to evaluate for the possibility of withdrawal and to improve pain management for patients who require additional medication. The timing of the assessment must be tailored to the patient's ability to communicate and participate, and to the patient's receptivity to the process. An assessment completed as soon as possible after injury may help the patient to make the connection between alcohol use and the injury.

Continuous assessment of the severity and extent of a person's injury is critical, as alcohol may complicate and lengthen the evaluation of the nature, extent, and severity of the injury.

Patients with traumatic injuries often present with an altered mental state, ranging from agitation and confusion to coma. The effect of alcohol can mimic the symptoms of traumatic brain injury; signs and symptoms may include behavior changes, sleepiness, and inappropriate language.

Accurate assessment also depends on whether the patient can feel tenderness or pain in response to touch. Alcohol can raise the pain threshold, thus decreasing a person's ability to feel pain. For example, an intoxicated patient with a cervical spine injury may report no tenderness in the neck and an individual with an internal injury may not feel pain.

Alcohol has a synergistic effect with a number of medications used for pain and sedation; these drugs acting together with alcohol can cause decreased blood pressure, slow respirations, or even apnea (temporary cessation of breathing). Alcohol often influences the choice of an anesthetic agent or its dose. Frequent, heavy use of alcohol enhances the ability of the liver to metabolize alcohol and other drugs. Thus, some anesthetics and other medications are cleared more quickly by the liver and the standard dose may give less than the expected effect or may result in a greater and more prolonged effect.

The Importance of ATOD Interventions in Injury

There is extensive evidence and wide agreement in the field that traumatic injury creates a "teachable moment" or a unique opportunity in the course of the addiction process (Reyna, Hollis, & Hulsebus, 1985; Soderstrom & Cowley, 1987). This teachable moment happens when a patient makes a connection in his or her mind that the traumatic injury is a direct result of alcohol and other drug use. Those who are able to make the connection may be more open to accepting education and treatment, greatly reducing their chances for reinjury and improving their course of recovery from the injury.

Assessing a patient can be approached in a variety of ways. Face to face assessment is a challenging and often difficult task, because of the denial that nearly always surrounds alcohol abuse problems. The health care provider should have a nonjudgmental, empathic attitude (Gentilello, Donovan, Dunn, & Rivara, 1995; Tweed, 1989). This is crucial to the success of this process. He or she should have an understanding about how to confront behaviors sometimes demonstrated by alcohol-dependent patients. The most direct method is to ask patients about their drinking habits as factually as you ask them about their allergies. You may be surprised by how open a response you can get with a nonjudgmental inquiry.

Many patients may fear participating in the assessment process because they may fear the result of the assessment will be obtained by the criminal justice system or that insurance companies will refuse to pay for treatment of injuries. The assessment process may be less threatening if the patient is assured that the results will be kept in the strictest confidence. (Specific information regarding the federal regulations governing confidentiality and redisclosure of ATOD information may be found in the Code of Federal Regulations Part 2 (42 C. F. R. Part 2), Confidentiality of Alcohol and Drug Abuse Patient Records.)

The assessment of trauma patients can be especially challenging. Traumatic injuries can complicate the alcohol assessment process in both physical and psychological ways. For example, patients may be unable to cooperate secondary to intubation, medications, and/or significant cognitive impairment. Psychologically, patients may be focused on the current crisis and be unwilling to shift their focus to talk about the alcohol problem. It is important to involve family members and other significant relations in the assessment (Beeder & Millman, 1992). Patients' families may provide vital information needed to plan care. It is important to note that the health care provider needs to be aware that the patient's family and friends may also use alcohol, consequently altering their responses.

Components of the Assessment

The components of an assessment consist of a complete medical and psychiatric history, including a mental status examination; a physical examination; a history of alcohol and other drug use; employment and support status; legal status, including involvement with the criminal justice system; educational history; family and social relationships; and financial status. The assessment should also take into account laboratory screening results.

Medical History

The medical history should include the family's medical history, including ATOD problems of parents, siblings, aunts, and uncles. The patient's trauma history should also be included. The Skinner Trauma History (Figure 6–4) consists of five questions about previous trauma injuries. A score of two or more positive responses to the five questions has been shown to indicate a high probability of excessive drinking or alcohol abuse (Keso, Kivisaari, & Salaspuro, 1988; Skinner et al., 1984). Obtaining the patient's trauma history is important because previous injuries are a primary predictor of future injury.

Additional elements of general medical history should include questions of previous episodes of hepatitis, infections, gastritis, and other instances of complications that frequently accompany alcohol dependence (Council on Mental Health, 1971).

Psychiatric History

The psychiatric history should include the history of alcohol use and treatment. Alcohol use and abuse problems are prevalent in individuals with psychiatric illness, although many psychiatric symptoms abate rapidly with abstinence. Providers should consider that alcohol may be an attempt to self-medicate psychiatric problems; the psychiatric disorder may be a consequence of the addiction; and addiction and psychiatric illness may develop in-

Since your 18th birthday
(1) Have you had any fractures or dislocations to your bones or joints?
(2) Have you been injured in a road traffic accident?
(3) Have you injured your head?
(4) Have you been injured in an assault or fight?
(5) Have you been injured after drinking?

FIGURE 6–4. Skinner Trauma History. (From "Identification of Alcohol Abuse Using Laboratory Tests and A History of Trauma," by H. A. Skinner, S. Holt, R. Schuller, J. Roy, & Y. Israell, 1984, *Annals of Internal Medicine, 101*, p. 848. Copyright 1984 by the American College of Physicians. Reprinted with permission.)

dependently and later impact on each other (Meyer, 1986; Senay, 1992). It is important to remember that the behavior of patients who have suffered brain injuries and the behavior of patients under the influence of drugs often mimic symptoms of psychiatric disorders and in some cases provoke them.

An initial psychiatric assessment may be completed, beginning with a determination of the potential risk of suicide or violence or the presence of psychosis. The purpose of psychiatric examination is to assess for threshold criteria of disorders requiring emergency intervention.

Risk Factors for Violence

- Stimulant or alcohol intoxication
- Psychotic states (drug induced or otherwise)
- Previous history of violent behaviors
- Availability of weapons
- History of childhood abuse (Kleber, 1994, p. 16)

Risk Factors for Suicide

- Age: 20–30
- Sex: Male
- Concurrent alcohol abuse and use of multiple substances, especially opioids, cocaine, amphetamines, sedatives
- Chronic use, including history of drug overdoses
- Stimulant withdrawal
- Comorbid psychiatric symptoms, especially depression, borderline personality disorder, psychoses, exhaustion
- Recent (within 6 weeks) significant loss
- Childhood history of hyperactivity, incorrigibility, family financial difficulties, family suicidal behaviors, abuse, living in foster homes
- Family history of depression, suicide, alcoholism
- Severe chronic pain (possibly) (Kleber, 1994, p. 16)

A full evaluation should proceed only after acute withdrawal and lingering withdrawal effects have passed (Dackis & Gold, 1992). The most common psychiatric disorders in this population are depression, anxiety, and antisocial behavior. As previously stated, psychiatric symptoms may be the result of agonist effects of drugs. However, psychiatric symptoms occurring after at least a 2–3 week period of abstinence are reliable indicators of psychiatric comorbidity (Beeder & Millman, 1992; Dackis & Gold, 1992).

One of the classification systems used to identify disorders related to psychoactive substance use is the *Diagnostic and Statistical Manual of Mental Disorders* (DSM-IV). It is beyond the scope of this book to describe the comorbid psychiatric disorders that may be present in the alcoholic.

ATOD History

In addition to a general medical history, a specific history must be sought, covering the introduction to alcohol and drugs and the development of abuse that led to the state of dependence. Information about patterns of alcohol and drug use can be obtained from the patient, family members, and significant others, and from physical signs and symptoms. Contemporary alcoholics frequently use other drugs (in descending frequency: nicotine, cannabis, cocaine, benzodiazepines, opiates, and hallucinogens (Kosten, Rounsaville, & Kleber, 1987; Miller & Gold, 1989). Therefore, clinical assessment and treatment must include consideration of other drugs in the history and laboratory testing, such as drug screens.

The ATOD history should include information from the following areas: precipitating events, previous attempts at treatment (dates, modalities, outcomes), onset of use, frequency of use, and duration and pattern of use (occasional versus regular). Include the period of heaviest use and the pattern of use within the past 3 weeks; periods of abstinence (number, duration, and circumstances); desired psychoactive effects; subjective and objective effects on the patient's physical, psychological, and emotional states; symptomatology of use for the patient, withdrawal symptomatology, and medical sequelae; list of all psychoactive drug(s) used and determination of age of onset; pattern of use and current status; and extent of social deterioration or isolation. This will assist in comprehending the interpersonal losses and the legal, educational, medical, and employment consequences the patient is facing (Beeder & Millman, 1992; Council on Mental Health, 1971).

Physical Examination

The physical examination should be performed with special emphasis on alcohol abnormalities. The patient's general appearance should be examined, as this can provide clues to the patient's self-perception (Alexander, Morello, Gould, & Peterson, 1993). A good assessment is the first step toward uncovering the hidden alcoholic (Table 6–1).

Table 6–1. Medical Findings Suggestive of Alcoholism.

Despite the tendency of alcoholics to deny or conceal their condition, the following may be utilized in assessing patients for physiological effects of alcohol abuse.

Signs	***Alcohol-Related Cause***
Central Nervous System	*Neurotoxicity*
❖ Unsteady gait	
❖ Unclear speech	
❖ Impaired cognitive ability	
❖ Memory loss, amnesiac periods	
❖ Cerebral atrophy	
❖ Stupor or coma	
❖ Neuropathies	
❖ Confusion	
❖ Confabulation	
❖ Subdural hematoma	
❖ Tremulousness	
❖ Slowed reflexes	Reflex depression
❖ Seizures	Hypoglycemia, possible hypomagnesemia Decreasing level of blood alcohol; lowers seizure threshold
❖ Sleep pattern deficits	Interference with REM and delta sleep
❖ Use of sedative or hypnotics	
❖ Tolerance to analgesics/alcohol	Nerve cell adaptation
Respiratory System	
❖ Chronic bronchitis	Alcohol-induced abnormalities in immune function
❖ Chronic obstructive pulmonary disease	
❖ Tuberculosis	
❖ Aspiration pneumonia	
Cardiovascular System	
❖ Cardiac arrhythmia	Vasodilation with decrease in peripheral resistance

Signs	***Alcohol-Related Cause***
Sinus tachycardia	
Atrial or nodal premature beats	Depressant effect of ethanol on myocardium
Ventricular premature beats	
Ventricular tachycardia	
❖ Cardiomyopathy	
❖ Refractory hypertension	
Gastrointestinal System	
❖ GI complaints	Irritation of mucous membranes
❖ Heavy use of antacids	Toxicity to GI mucosa, causing inflammation and edema
❖ Carcinoma	
❖ Esophageal varices	Increased gastric secretions
❖ Gastritis	
❖ Abdominal tenderness	
❖ Parotid gland enlargement	
❖ Peptic ulcers	
❖ Decreased hemoglobin/hematocrit	GI bleeding
❖ Pernicious anemia (folic acid deficiency)	GI malabsorption
❖ Fissures at corner of mouth; smooth red tongue	Vitamin deficiency
❖ Pancreatitis (acute or chronic)	Toxicity to pancreatic cells
❖ Type II diabetes	Pancreatic duct obstruction from edema of intestinal mucosa
❖ Elevated liver enzymes, elevated bilirubin	Hepatotoxicity, possibly leading to hepatitis, cirrhosis
❖ Low BUN	Liver gives priority to metabolism impairing other functions
❖ High serum ammonia	
❖ High amylase	
❖ Electrolyte imbalances	
❖ Cirrhosis	
❖ Hepatitis	
❖ Enlarged or tender liver; ascites	
❖ Distended jugular veins	
❖ Spider nevi	Impaired portal circulation
❖ Elevated blood sugar	Impaired sugar metabolism
❖ Thiamine deficiency	Liver stores exhausted during metabolism
❖ Niacin deficiency	
Hematologic System	
❖ Abnormal RBC morphology	Bone marrow toxicity
❖ Abnormal RBC volumes	Nutritional deficiencies
❖ Decreased hemoglobin or hematocrit	Splenic enlargement
❖ Increased MCV (mean corpuscular volume)	
❖ Anemia	
❖ Decreased platelet count	Impaired platelet production

(continued)

Table 6–1. *(continued)*

Endocrine System	
❖ Increased urinary output	Diuresis from decrease in hypothalamic production
❖ Dehydration	of antidiuretic hormone as blood alcohol rises
❖ Decreased urinary output	As blood alcohol drops, impaired
❖ Edema, "puffy" face	hypothalamus may oversecrete antidiuretic hormone
Hyperglycemia	Impaired pituitary function disrupts
❖ Hypoglycemia	insulin production
❖ "Dirty tan" skin color	Impaired pituitary function disrupts melancoyte-stimulating hormone
❖ Decreased sexual desire	Impaired hypothalamic/pituitary/
❖ Infertility	gonadal axis effects testosterone, estrogen levels.
❖ Men:	
Gynecomastia	
Decreased facial hair	
Impotence	
❖ Women:	
Lack of vaginal lubrication	
Irregular menstruation, amenorrhea	
Genitourinary System	
❖ Gout (increased blood uric acid)	Impaired kidney acid excretion
❖ Frequent urinary tract infections	Urinary retention
❖ Prostatitis	Tissue toxicity
❖ Testicular atrophy	Decreased testosterone synthesis
Skin/Muscular Skeletal System	
❖ Fractures (especially ribs)	Compromised judgment
❖ Burns, especially 3rd degree	Reduced sensory-motor control
❖ Lacerations	Slowed reflexes
❖ Cigarette stains on fingers	Impaired cognitive function
❖ Freezing or cold injury	
❖ Other accidents: scars; infections	
❖ Muscle weakness	Toxicity to muscle cells
❖ Decreased muscle mass	Anemia
❖ Peripheral neuropathies	Thiamine deficiency

Sources: Fleming, M. F., & Barry, K. L. (1992). *Addictive disorders.* St Louis: Mosby-Year Book, Inc.; Luckmann, J., & Sorensen, K. C. (1974). *Medical-surgical nursing-A psychophysiologic approach.* Philadelphia: W.B. Suanders Company; Ray, O., & Ksir, C. (1993). *Drugs, society, and human behavior* (6th ed.). St. Louis, MO: Mosby-Year Book, Inc.; Roselle, G. A. (1992). Alcohol and the immune system. *Alcohol Health & Research, 16,* 16–22.

The patient should be examined in the following way: the head for contusions, fractures, abrasions, and wounds on the skull caused by falls and accidents; the eyes for red conjunctiva and jaundiced sclera; the skin for flushing and diaphoresis associated with intoxication and withdrawal; the breath for odor of alcohol; and verbalizations for slurred speech, inappropriate responses, contradictory replies, evasion, long rambling stories, memory lapses, emotional lability (especially anger and tears), irritability, confusion, anxiety, depression, guilt, suicidal ideation, and lethargy.

Other indicators include fractured ribs or bruises from falls; a history of pulmonary and/or cardiovascular problems; a protruding abdomen (beer belly), an enlarged liver, and peripheral edema; systemic jaundice; history of diagnosed fatty liver or cirrhosis; history of gastritis, hemoptysis, pancreatitis, malabsorption syndrome and/or ulcers; colitis; signs of dehydration and malnutrition; complaints of nausea, vomiting, anorexia, and diarrhea.

In addition, fractures and wounds at various stages of healing, circulatory and neurological deficits, weakness, dermatitis, pruritus, ataxia, fine or gross tremors (or shakes), and muscle spasms associated with intoxication or withdrawal are also indicators of alcohol abuse. Muscle wasting is a sign of advanced alcoholism, usually seen in those who have been drinking for decades. Since dental neglect is common among alcoholics, inspect teeth carefully. Check the body for signs of liver impairment such as spider angiomata, and jaundice. Evaluate the nervous system carefully for signs of cerebral and cerebellar atrophy and peripheral neuropathy. Finally, inspect the skin for gooseflesh, purpura, petechiae, and spider nevi—the so-called W. C. Fields nose (Alexander et al., 1993).

It is important to remember that today it is more common than not to have an individual abusing alcohol in combination with other drugs. When conducting a physical assessment you must be alert to signs indicative of other types of drug use.

Behavior

The last and the most difficult area to assess is behavior. Look for any change in behavior or level of consciousness. Notable behaviors to watch for are nervousness, anxiety, restlessness, irritability, hyperexcitability, insomnia, paranoia, lethargy, and depression. Is there evidence of memory loss, suicidal or homicidal ideation, difficulty concentrating, secretive or isolative behaviors, or low pain tolerance? Any or all of these symptoms are red flags and require further investigation (Alexander et al., 1993).

Other clues are some common admission diagnoses: new onset seizures, aspiration pneumonia, physical trauma, motor vehicle accidents, gastritis, hepatitis, and pancreatitis, as well as cirrhosis and gastrointestinal bleeding. Burns, frostbite, cellulitis, and old untreated injuries (e.g., broken ribs), all could be associated with alcohol dependency. Recurrent illness without any other explainable cause also can be indicators (Alexander et al., 1993).

This is by no means an all-inclusive list. When interviewing and working with patients, health care professionals often get an indication of difficulties in the home as well as problems on the job, and spiritual bankruptcy. These can all be indications of alcohol dependency.

Postassessment Considerations

Because alcoholics often deny that they have problems, the health care professional should present and discuss the results of the assessment. In early interactions, avoid using words that label the patient, such as alcoholic. Such terms can increase the patient's denial and evoke a defensive response. Patients respond to cues in voice and manner that reveal the feelings and attitudes of the provider.

The essential elements in a relationship with an alcoholic patient are knowledge about the disease, a nonjudgmental attitude, and the ability to confront an individual with alcohol dependence with the same professional acceptance that one would adopt toward a patient with any other disease. The patient must be treated with respect and consideration. To establish trust and confidence, the health care professional must answer the patient's questions about his or her health and care honestly and completely.

By addressing the patient by name, making eye contact, and encouraging patient decision-making, the health care professional demonstrates sincere interest in promoting the patient's self-esteem and sense of well-being. An essential tool in successful treatment is respect for the patient as a unique person who can be helped, but who must be allowed the dignity of choice.

It is important to recognize that the patient must admit that there may be a connection between the use of alcohol and problems in living before he or she will accept assistance. It may be more beneficial to focus on the problems in everyday living caused by the alcohol than concentrating solely on the behaviors. A broad open-ended clarifying statement may elicit the patient's willingness to look at the problem. Asking a "why" question often blocks communication. The plans for treatment or referral should be personal, supportive, specific, and action-oriented and be mutually agreed upon by the patient and health care professional.

SUMMARY

Awareness and recognition are the clinician's best tools in preventing withdrawal from alcohol and the concomitant medical complications. Clinicians should prepare themselves to be aware of many factors in order to prevent complication, provide better patient care, and educate patients and families.

Once the initial assessment is completed, a realistic withdrawal prevention plan can be developed. To do so, one must be aware of the resources that are available in each institution, as well as in the community. These may include desk references such as standards of care and resource books on the care of the alcohol-dependent patient, access to a consultation service, and a unit-based treatment team, to name a few.

The diagnosis of dependence is based primarily on history, physical examination, and clinical observations. Diagnosis is usually not difficult. Frequently, the patient admits dependence. Even so, an adequate history must be procured to substantiate the patient's statements and to determine and assess the degree of dependence, patterns of use, and motivation (Council on Mental Health, 1971).

Once the diagnosis is confirmed, the health care professional should inform the patient of the effects of alcohol and should develop a plan that is tailored to the needs of the patient.

CHAPTER 7

TREATMENT OF ALCOHOL WITHDRAWAL

❖ **Pharmacological Interventions**
❖ **Additional Considerations**

On initial assessment, symptoms of withdrawal can mimic or overlap with symptoms of injury, confusing the immediate clinical picture. Patients experiencing alcohol withdrawal frequently become agitated, which is highly dangerous in some trauma situations, especially in a spinal cord injury. Unrecognized withdrawal states, such as alcohol withdrawal, can lead to delirium tremens, a dangerous and sometimes fatal condition, if left untreated, especially after surgery. Because of the potential of this situation, it is imperative that alcohol withdrawal be addressed as soon as possible.

The clinical assessment of alcohol withdrawal is largely guided by vital signs and patient appearance. Virtually anyone, whether tolerant to alcohol or not, will show an elevation in blood pressure and pulse after low doses of alcohol. Because vital signs are objective and reliable indicators of alcohol withdrawal, frequent monitoring will usually reveal the severity of withdrawal.

PHARMACOLOGICAL INTERVENTIONS

Initial management should provide fluid, electrolyte, and vitamin supplementation as needed. Mild symptoms can be managed with a quiet, supportive environment, reorientation, and one-to-one contact. If patients progress symptomatically despite a supportive environment, pharmacologic treatment should be instituted. Since alcohol withdrawal affects many neurotransmitter and neuroendocrine systems, numerous drugs have been tried to treat it (Nutt & Glue, 1990; Wilkens & Gorelick, 1986). For inpatients experiencing moderate to severe alcohol withdrawal, the most widely accepted pharmacotherapy for withdrawal symptoms is the prophylactic use of benzodiazepines (Charness, Simon, & Greenberg, 1989; Naranjo & Sellers, 1986). They are effective for most withdrawal symptoms and safe even at high doses. They carry minimal risk of drug-drug interactions, which is especially important for patients hospitalized with concomitant medical conditions.

Propranolol and clonidine, which reduce the overactivity of adrenergic neurons, are used to treat symptoms of severe tremor or cardiac arrhythmias (Charness et al., 1989; Naranjo & Sellers, 1986). Antipsychotic drugs that are less likely to cause sedation or hypotension or induce seizures are administered to control hallucinations (Charness et al., 1989; Naranjo & Sellers, 1986).

Treatment of withdrawal is designed to suppress the abstinence withdrawal by consecutive dose reduction (tapering) with the same drug or with one with similar pharmacologic properties. Typically, one drug is preferred over another in detoxification because of pharmacokinetic properties such as route and rate of absorption and elimination half-life (the time required to eliminate half the concentration of a drug).

Benzodiazepines. Benzodiazepines have remained the mainstay in the treatment of alcohol withdrawal since their introduction in the 1960s. All benzodiazepines are similar in their pharmacodynamic properties by their specific action at the GABA receptor. They differ only in their absorption, elimination time, and production of active metabolites. The intermediate acting drugs (24–36 hours) such as chlordiazepoxide (Librium) and diazepam (Valium) are preferred to minimize fluctuating blood levels. Shorter acting drugs (6–12 hours) such as lorazepam (Ativan) and alprazolam (Xanax) are less desirable because of the intensification of withdrawal symptoms. Studies have shown that benzodiazepines are effective in suppressing and preventing signs and symptoms of withdrawal, including seizures and delirium tremens. However, they are only effective if the principle of giving enough to induce initially sustained mild intoxication followed by gradual reduction of the daily dosage is followed.

Medication treatment choices and dosage depend on alcohol history, age, and health status of the patient, metabolism factors, and treatment drug half-life. Impaired hepatic function can prolong drug half-life, increasing the risk of oversedation. To minimize this danger, give only enough medication to make the patient comfortable and keep the pulse rate down.

It is important to review the following information: Chlordiazepoxide (Librium) or diazepam (Valium) are the benzodiazepines most often used. Lorazepam (Ativan) is the only benzodiazepine with reliable intramuscular absorption, and if active metabolites are of concern in patients with hepatic or renal compromise, oxazepam (Serax) or lorazepam, which do have not active metabolites, should be prescribed. Finally, in a hospital setting, prescribing benzodiazepines on an as-needed (p.r.n.) basis is not advisable (Sees, 1991).

Nursing personnel, given p.r.n. only orders, face the task of deciding when a patient really needs the medication and when the patient is drug seeking, or when the medication is being dispensed to quiet an "obnoxious patient." Instead, it is better to write an around-the-clock dose of the benzodiazepine at the estimated (or slightly less than the estimated) need of the patient for 24 hours. In addition to the around-the-clock order, a hold order should be included for the patient who is sleeping or appears somnolent at the time the next dose is due, as well as a qualified p.r.n. order for additional benzodiazepines. The use of medication should be reviewed daily and the orders adjusted as needed. The benzodiazepines are tapered over an average of 3 to 7 days (Sees, 1991).

Anticonvulsants. The severity of withdrawal symptoms tends to increase progressively in alcoholics who have undergone repeated episodes of withdrawal (Brown, Anton, Malcom, & Ballenger, 1988). This phenomenon may be comparable to a form of brain sensitization called *kindling*—small electrical currents, individually too small to produce a seizure, will ultimately produce a seizure if applied repeatedly (Ballenger & Post, 1978). Therefore, medications that inhibit kindling, such as anticonvulsants, have been examined for treating alcohol withdrawal.

Pentobarbital (Luminal) is very effective and can be used in withdrawal, particularly in patients with a history of seizures either from alcohol withdrawal or other causes. An added advantage of phenobarbital is its cross-tolerance and dependence with alcohol in suppressing the full spectrum of the alcohol withdrawal syndrome. However, disadvantages are the long half-life and, therefore, prolonged clearance and potentially synergistic effect with other sedating drugs.

Long-acting barbiturates such as phenobarbital may be preferred in alcohol withdrawal patients with increased cranial pressure. These drugs are cross-tolerant with alcohol and possess anticonvulsant activity. Compared to benzodiazepines, however, there is greater risk of respiratory and central nervous system depression, and the ability of barbiturates to induce hepatic enzymes presents a greater potential for interactions with medications.

Carbamazepine (Tegretol) has been reported effective in treatment of alcohol withdrawal as well as barbiturates. There are advantages to using a barbiturate for alcohol withdrawal: they are long acting and therefore can be dosed infrequently, they are seizure protective, and their abuse potential is low. However, there are also disadvantages: they have a narrow therapeutic index, therefore, the difference between a dose needed to control withdrawal symptoms and a toxic dose may be very small, and they may interfere with other medications (Sees, 1991).

Beta Blockers. Other medications for use in alcohol withdrawal are beta blockers, which are useful for controlling blood pressure and tachyarrhythmias, as well as for decreasing tremors more quickly (Guthrie, 1989). In addition, a combination of beta blockers and a benzodiazepine more effectively treats alcohol withdrawal, and according to Zilm and colleagues (1980), fewer benzodiazepines are needed. However, it is important to note that beta blockers may increase hypoglycemia, induce bronchospasm, decrease cardiac functioning, compromise breathing in patients with chronic obstructive pulmonary disease (Sees, 1991), and increase the incidence of hallucinations during alcohol withdrawal. Also, they do not prevent progression to more serious withdrawal symptoms, do not relieve anxiety, and have no effect on seizures (Guthrie, 1989). It is therefore recommended that, when beta blockers are used for treating alcohol withdrawal, they be combined with a benzodiazepine or a barbiturate (Sees, 1991).

Clonidine. Clonidine is also used for alcohol detoxification. It controls tachycardia and hypertension (Manhem, Nilsson, Moberg, Wadstein, & Hokfelt, 1985), and also provides symptomatic relief by decreasing anxiety, tremor, tension, nausea, vomiting, palpitations, restlessness, diaphoresis, and depression (Walinder, Balldin, Bokstrom, Karlsson, & Lundstrom, 1981). Other advantages to clonidine are that: there is both an oral and transdermal form of the medication; it is not a psychoactive dependence-producing medication; and it is not a controlled substance. However, it has not been shown to be more effective than benzodiazepines. Also, it is not cross-tolerant with alcohol and its use is limited to mild cases, as it is inadequate alone for moderate symptoms and may mask progression to severe withdrawal.

Buspirone (Buspar). Buspirone is also receiving considerable attention for treating alcohol withdrawal symptoms (Bruno, 1989; Tollefson, 1992). Compared with benzodiazepines, buspirone produces little if any sedation, which may enable patients to participate in rehab more readily during the first few days of alcohol withdrawal. Other advantages are that: tolerance does not develop; there is no withdrawal when it is discontinued, even if discontinued abruptly; it produces no euphoria; and there appears to be no reinforcement for self-medication or self-dosing (Anton, 1994; Sees, 1991). In addition, current research suggests that buspirone may be helpful in alleviating the psychological symptoms that accompany alcoholism (Malec, Malec, Gagné, & Dongier, 1996). It is recommended that buspirone not be used in patients with a history of alcohol withdrawal seizures or in patients who are concurrently using benzodiazepines and/or barbiturates.

Magnesium. Magnesium can be used to increase the seizure threshold if the magnesium level is low. If, however, the initial magnesium level is normal, magnesium supplementation has probably little associated benefit. In addition, renal function must be normal before magnesium supplementation can be considered.

ADDITIONAL CONSIDERATIONS

When considering alcohol withdrawal, it is important to remember vitamin supplementation. Most important is thiamine; WKS can be avoided (Clark, Sees, & Nathan, 1988). Other vitamin supplementation depends on the patient's nutritional status, but those most frequently added are folic acid, iron, a multivitamin, and vitamin K if the partial thromboplastin time is prolonged. Toxicity of vitamin supplementation must also be considered (Clark et al., 1988).

SUMMARY

Once established, alcoholism has the characteristics of a chronic, relapsing disorder. Periodic withdrawal is accomplished by many alcoholics even without medical assistance, but repeated relapse to alcohol use is common, and the duration of periods of abstinence usually is short (Council on Mental Health, 1971).

CHAPTER 8

CONVENTIONAL TREATMENT APPROACHES TO ALCOHOL DEPENDENCY

- **Treatment Components**
- **Treatment Settings**
- **Relapse Prevention Strategies**

During the past decade treatment options have grown dramatically. Health care professionals are finding new ways to deal with old issues. The patient must now make choices. To the alcohol-dependent patient, the option is always there to stop drinking. Even deep in the throes of addiction, the option is always there. Yet choosing to quit requires such a monumental effort, it is very much as if the individual chooses a new life. The life of recovery begins with one choice, the choice not to drink. Additionally, other choices need to be made, choices concerning this new lifestyle. Of course, the more these other choices support recovery, the more likely it is that the individual will succeed.

One of the first things to understand about treating alcoholism is: There *is* no cure for alcoholism. But it *is* treatable, and can be arrested. Alcoholism has long been recognized as a chronic relapsing disorder; even if an alcoholic has not taken a drink for years, that person is still referred to as "recovering," not "recovered." This is because the potential for relapse always exists and staying sober requires a continuing lifelong effort (National Institutes of Health [NIH], 1993).

Among programs in the treatment field, 12-step support groups have the longest history and, for a period of time, this type of program became the most widely recommended. Indeed, it may still may be the most popular program in the field today. However, 12-step groups are not for everyone. That is why it is important that professionals be aware of available treatment options. The one-size-fits-all idea has finally given way to the more realistic idea that people are different and can benefit from different types of interventions. The patient's choice of treatment should be included in discharge and aftercare planning.

TREATMENT COMPONENTS

To begin the rehabilitation, the patient must be willing to participate in the process. Of course patients may refuse treatment, but the decision must be theirs to make. Health care providers should not assume that it is useless to offer therapy, even if it has been refused in the past.

Once the initial phase of treatment is instituted and the withdrawal signs and symptoms have been prevented or controlled, it is time to plan for recovery. Just as with any other classification of patient, discharge planning begins with the initial assessment. Alcohol-dependent patients will require much supportive therapy. Part of this therapy must be instituted while they are inpatients. They should be provided with a supportive learning environment and a well-defined aftercare plan that includes the family and significant others in interventions whenever possible.

Spontaneous Recovery

Not everyone needs treatment to be successful. In fact, the number of individuals who enter recovery on their own (known as "spontaneous recovery") has been proven in studies to be significant (Bufe, 1991).

Indeed, according to a scientific survey, professional help has little to do with important life changes, even health-related ones. Physicians helped people change only 3% of the time—and psychologists and psychiatrists, self-help groups, and religious counselors received the credit even less often. Support was much more likely to come from friends (14%), parents, children, or siblings (21%), or a spouse, boyfriend, or girlfriend (29%). And 30% of the time, individuals simply did what they had to do on their own (Gurion, 1990).

In other research, focused specifically on alcoholism, findings suggest that "20% of alcoholics can and do quit successfully on their own." (Neimark, Conway, & Doskoch, 1994)

The first step of alcoholism treatment is managing the signs and symptoms of withdrawal (refer to Chapter 7). Following this, treatment is initiated. The majority of treatment components strive to achieve long-term abstinence or reduce alcohol consumption in patients. Components that show particular promise for effective treatment fall into two broad categories. One category consists of strategies to reduce alcohol use directly, such as brief interventions, pharmacotherapy, behavioral self-control training, and cue extinction. The second category includes strategies to reduce alcohol use indirectly through enhancement of social and coping skills (e.g., behavioral marital therapy, relapse prevention, and stress management) (Miller, 1992).

Brief Interventions

Growing evidence now indicates that brief interventions are effective in decreasing alcohol use by heavy drinkers who are not yet physically dependent on alcohol (Institute of Medicine, 1990a). Physicians and other health care professionals deliver these interventions based on an assessment of the patient's alcohol use and alcohol-related problems. During a brief, highly directive consultation, the professional informs the patient about the assessment results (e.g., elevated liver functions, absenteeism or lateness at work, or alcohol-related arrests). The professional then offers clear strategies, such as goal setting and contracting, to reduce future drinking.

Pharmacotherapy for Inhibiting Drinking Behaviors

Two general maintenance treatment approaches have evolved to treat the addictive behaviors from alcohol. First is maintenance treatment, that substitutes the addicting substance with a cross-tolerant and dependent drug. These drugs are sometimes referred to as *agonists*. The second advocates maintenance treatment with an *antagonist* drug that blocks the effects of the addicting drug by occupying the same receptor sites in the brain (Sees, 1991).

Three types of medications have been researched on the long-term treatment of alcohol abuse/dependence: anticraving drugs, alcohol sensitizing drugs, and drugs that treat concurrent psychiatric disorders.

Anticraving Medications

Naltrexone. Naltrexone, an opiate antagonist considered to be an anticraving medication, has recently been approved by the Food and Drug Administration as a treatment for alcoholism. Unlike disulfiram, which is discussed later, naltrexone is not used as an aversive therapy and does not cause an Antabuse-like reaction, either as a result of opiate use or ethanol ingestion. In preliminary studies, the opiate antagonist appears to reduce the frequency of relapse (Greenstein, Fudala, & O'Brien 1992; O'Malley et al., 1992; Ried, Delconte, Nichols, Bilsky, & Hubbell, 1991; Ried & Hunter, 1984; Volpicelli, Davis, & Olfin, 1986; Volpicelli, O'Brien, Alterman, & Hayashida, 1990; Wesson & Ling, 1991). Currently, NIAAA is funding nine additional clinical trials to determine the patient type, dose, therapy combinations, and treatment duration with which naltrexone works best.

Questions and Answers About Naltrexone Treatment for Alcoholism

1. What is naltrexone?

Naltrexone is a medication that blocks the effects of opioids by competing for opioid receptors in the brain. It was originally used to treat dependence on opioid drugs but has recently been approved by the FDA as a treatment for alcoholism.

2. **Why does naltrexone help alcoholism?**
   Although the precise mechanism of action for naltrexone's effect is unknown, reports from successfully treated patients suggest three kinds of effects: it reduces cravings, helps patients remain abstinent, and interferes with the tendency to want to drink more if a recovering patient slips and has a drink.
3. **Is naltrexone a stand-alone treatment for alcoholism?**
   No, naltrexone is only one component of a comprehensive treatment program.
4. **How long does naltrexone take to work?**
   Naltrexone's effects occur shortly after taking the first dose.
5. **Who should not take naltrexone?**
   Naltrexone should not be used with pregnant women, individuals with severe liver or kidney damage, or with patients who cannot achieve abstinence for at least 5 days prior to initiating medications.
6. **What does it feel like to be on naltrexone?**
   Aside from mild side effects, patients usually report that they are largely unaware of being on the medication.
7. **What are the side effects of naltrexone?**
   The most common side effects of naltrexone include the following: nausea, headache, dizziness, fatigue, insomnia, anxiety, and sleepiness. These side effects are usually mild and of short duration.
8. **How do you manage pain in patients maintained on naltrexone?**
   Because naltrexone is an opioid blocker, it may inhibit the effectiveness of opioid analgesics which are administered for the purposes of managing pain. In patients maintained on naltrexone, when possible, nonopioid pain medications or approaches should be tried first. Thus, the use of nonsteroidal anti-inflammatory agents should be considered as first-line pharmacological therapy for pain management. In situations where opioids are necessary for the treatment of severe pain the following approach should be taken. The blockade can be overridden with a rapidly acting analgesic, but treatment requires close monitoring in a setting equipped and staffed for cardiopulmonary resuscitation because the resulting respiratory depression may be deeper and more prolonged.

Benzodiazepines. Benzodiazepines and their agonists have not been extensively studied as a substitution for alcohol because clinical and research experience shows alcoholic relapse to alcohol while on benzodiazepines. Moreover, benzodiazepines themselves are addicting and produce significant pharmacologic tolerance and dependence (Miller & Gold, 1989, 1991).

Bromocriptine. Bromocriptine (Parlodel), a dopamine agonist, has theoretical rationale because of its direct action on dopamine receptors.

Buspirone. In an 8-week trial, buspirone (BuSpar) diminished alcohol craving, anxiety, and depression when administered to mild to moderate alcoholics. More research is needed to suggest utility in clinical practice (Bruno, 1989).

Aversive Agents

Aversive agents are designed to establish a pattern of avoidance, producing unpleasant reactions when combined with alcohol. Their use is sometimes referred to as deterrent therapy (Sees, 1991).

Disulfiram. The major aversive agent to alcohol has been disulfiram (Antabuse), an alcohol-sensitizing medication that is used to discourage patients from drinking during their rehabilitation. When combined with alcohol, disulfiram inhibits the enzyme acetaldehyde dehydrogenase, causing the ethanol byproduct acetaldehyde to build up, producing unpleasant effects. Antabuse usually causes these effects, with diminishing intensity, for 4–5 days. In the presence of disulfiram alcohol consumption produces an accumulation of acetaldehyde, which can cause headache, diaphoresis, nausea and vomiting, facial flushing, increased blood pressure and heart rate, cardiovascular collapse, seizures, and death.

Controlled studies have shown Antabuse to be an effective treatment approach to alcohol dependence as long as the patient continues to take it (Azrin, Sisson, Meyers, & Godley, 1982; Fuller et al., 1986).

It is important to note that disulfiram produces a chronic toxicity that appears to be related both to dose and duration. Hepatitis, peripheral neuropathy, and sexual dysfunction have also been reported in chronic use of disulfiram.

Other examples of alcohol-sensitizing medications include calcium carbimide and daidzin (Anton, 1994). Because of significant toxic effects on the liver, their use in clinical practice is not recommended.

Psychiatric Medications

A number of studies have demonstrated an association between alcoholism and other psychiatric disorders, such as anxiety. Alcoholism may predispose an individual to a variety of psychiatric disorders. Conversely, some psychiatric disturbances may contribute to the development of alcoholism and further exacerbate the primary mental disorder (Liskow & Goodwin, 1987).

Because alcoholism is sometimes associated with cyclothymic disorder—a milder course of manic-depressive illness—lithium has been tried in alcoholics, but research studies showed no clear effectiveness (Fawcett et al., 1984; Merry, Reynolds, Bailey, & Coppen, 1976).

More recently, researchers have studied medications that reduce the uptake of the neurochemical serotonin (e.g., fluoxetine [Prozac] or zimelidine) (Anton, 1994). These drugs have known antidepressant properties and also decrease food and fluid consumption; either mechanism could decrease alcohol use.

Marital/Family Therapy

Couples or family therapy identifies family system issues linked to both the patient's alcohol use and to enabling behavior that promotes continued use. This approach provides support and education for the family, helps heal damage done by the patient's alcoholism, and reduces interpersonal difficulties and dysfunctional interactions that promote relapse.

Within family systems, alcoholic behavior has a purpose, and it is important to assess this. Family therapy is usually not sufficient as the sole means of treatment for alcoholism. Rather, it is a valuable and often essential adjunct to other treatment components (Doweiko, 1993; Institute of Medicine, 1990b; McCrady et al., 1986; Zweben, Pearlman, & Li, 1988).

Alcohol and Codependency

Those closest to the alcohol-dependent person are probably the first to feel the impact of the disease, yet as they adapt to survive the addictive system, are usually the last to be treated or considered in the treatment process. This is particularly unfortunate, because the dependent person will find it difficult to live productively with sobriety when the family members who have learned to live with addiction continue to operate in the same patterns as before sobriety.

Family Systems

The family is a system that seeks to protect its integrity and ensure its continuance through adaptation to stressful events and changing conditions. In alcoholic families, this often means that other members of the family, or "codependents," adapt to the family malfunction and to the alcoholic's disease, getting "sick" themselves in the process. This assuming of responsibility for the alcoholic's behavior "enables" the alcoholic to continue drinking (Whitfield, 1984).

Indicators of alcohol-related problems within a family system include quarrels over drinking, physical abuse, decreased socialization with friends, history of divorce, withdrawal of children, family history of alcoholism, abstinence, broken homes, children leaving home; and financial worries.

Codependency has been defined as being dependent on another's moods and behaviors, basing self-esteem on compulsive use of survival tactics, and generally measuring well-being on the status of a relationship. Family members experience the same compulsion, delusion, and denial seen in the alcoholic.

It is easy to identify codependency if you listen. Codependents will share with you all they have done or feel they should do. They may come to you in fear, questioning what they did or should have done to change their loved one's drinking. They have gradually compromised their own value system and what they want in their lives, and it may be difficult for them to see that they need to or can change.

Some of the clues in recognizing codependency include: rambling on about insignificant subjects or events when you address the drinking; explaining extensively what the alcoholic did, said, will do next; blaming the job, family, parents, and so on; letting you know how wonderful the alcoholic is, or what has been put up with for years. Most of their conversation will center on the alcoholic's behavior.

Codependents' behavior can be changed to the degree that the family members are willing to take risks. To do this, they need information on alcoholism and family choices and they need to know that they are dealing with an illness that they did not cause and one they cannot cure. Information will help them understand the disease and alleviate some of their guilt and frustration when trying to change the alcoholic. Most find it difficult to relinquish control, so if they are not ready to face the challenges, honor their choice.

If they are prepared, help them see how and why their reactions have proven unsuccessful. Define in simple terms the roles they may have assumed in an attempt to alleviate pain. Give them examples that they can relate to and, if possible, use their own examples. Show them how normal their reaction is. Honor and acknowledge the strength of what they have been doing, while showing them how to use their strengths to get their needs met. Address the issue of feelings by helping them cut through denials that may or may not be real. Honest feedback or confrontation may be helpful and therapeutic, if done without judgment.

You may also suggest that they participate in support group activities. Most codependents respond well to other codependents through common feelings, defenses, and choices, and begin to form a support system. Sometimes codependents need to be let go and allowed to learn by experience, after which they will be more receptive to new directions.

Recovery and Families

The process of recovery involves families moving away from neglecting their own needs, beliefs, and values, and trying to stop fixing, controlling, or being accepted by others. The family needs to develop several areas to move through recovery—awareness, insight, knowledge of defenses, enabling behaviors, and hidden emotions; each of which should be addressed through the help of 12-step programs. Old roles and negative emotions must be discarded and new attitudes chosen that promote well-being and personal growth, helping them to evaluate their self-worth and progress into healthy, functioning people.

Coping Skills Training

The coping skills training approach to alcoholism treatment addresses a patient's behavioral deficits, responses to antecedents, and the consequences of drinking. Training is based primarily on principles of social learning theory, which considers cognitive, environmental, and behavioral factors (Abrams & Niaura, 1987). The emphasis is on teaching or enhancing the skills required for achieving abstinence and for coping with the problems of daily life that could lead to drinking.

Self-Control Training

This approach focuses on what patients can do to modify their own behavior. It includes identifying drinking situations, setting goals, monitoring oneself, learning and practicing coping skills, and rewarding oneself for accomplishing goals (Hester & Miller, 1989). Patients can receive guidance from a clinician or a self-help manual.

Aversion Therapy

This approach involves pairing stressful or painful stimuli with actual alcohol consumption or pairing images of drinking with images of unpleasant scenes or experiences (Rimmele, Miller, & Dougher, 1989).

Cue Exposure Therapy

Environmental stimuli may play an important role in alcohol abuse. They can become associated with either the positive or aversive properties of alcohol (Siegel, 1989; Stewart & Eikelboom, 1987). These conditioned cues can profoundly affect the strength or weakness of alcohol-seeking behavior, physiological responses, and subjective states.

This therapy uses repeated exposure to stimuli to help the patient master the experience without drinking. The patient is helped to find a substitute image to counter the craving experience, until he or she reports no more craving when exposed to that stimulus (Cooney, Baker, & Ponerleau, 1983; Mansfield & Cunningham, 1980; Melchoir & Tavakoff, 1981). The more authentic the stimulus is to the patient's experience, the more effective the technique.

Motivational Interviewing

This approach has been developed to enhance patient motivation (Miller & Rollnick, 1991). Its goal is to help patients resolve their ambivalence and reach a commitment to change.

Motivational interviewing starts with the clinician recognizing and accepting patient ambivalence. Proceeding through what may be characterized as a gradual shaping process, the clinician tries to move the patient toward acknowledging his or her current problems, developing a desire to change them, and identifying strategies that will enable this change (Shaffer & Robbins, 1995).

Psychoeducation

Psychoeducation is a process of presenting information to patients and their families about addiction and then discussing individual attitudes and feelings toward alcohol use. When used with other treatment approaches, psychoeducation may increase patients' ability to function independently and meet their daily living needs outside the hospital setting (Stark & Campbell, 1991).

When developing a psychoeducational program, introduce the program at the beginning of hospitalization if possible. Be sure to adapt educational materials to the patient's level of understanding and language. Components of the program may include discussion of assumptions regarding alcohol; discussion about sexual behaviors and how they can trigger relapses to alcohol use; provision of psychoeducational material to families of alcoholics to provide guidance in how to support recovery efforts; and discussion of the power of triggers and how they relate to relapse (Stark & Campbell, 1991).

An educational program that helps the significant other and/or family members identify and understand the behaviors that encourage and support drinking can have a significant effect, often encouraging drinkers to enter treatment and to reduce their drinking (Thomas, Yoshioka, & Ager, 1996).

Psychotherapy

Psychotherapy focuses on intrapsychic processes that impair effective coping and damage relationships, while counseling historically has focused on external issues relating to the patient's life problems (Rounsaville & Carroll, 1992; Woody, McLellan, Luborsky, & O'Brien, 1990; Zweben, 1993).

Behavior Modification

This is generally used in treatment to suppress patients' negative behavior and reward positive behavior. In this sense, the behavioral intervention takes the form of rules and regulations about standards of behavior while in treatment and includes actions for rule breaking (Woody, McLellan, Luborsky, & O'Brien, 1985).

Contingency Contracting

Contingency contracting, also commonly referred to as contingency management, is a way to reinforce desired behavior by providing immediate consequences. This approach is useful as it sets concrete goals and emphasizes positive behavior change.

TREATMENT SETTINGS

Residential and Nonresidential Programs: Therapeutic Communities, Hospitals, and Self-Help Groups

Therapeutic Communities

Therapeutic communities (TCs) are full-time, highly structured, 1 to 2 year, drug-free residential programs phasing into independent residence with continuing contact for a period of time. These communities are highly organized and provide peer support, counseling, and residential job functions. Originally designed to provide structure and a productive environment for individuals (Institute of Medicine, 1990b), today TCs have broadened the methods they use. Almost all have retained group sessions, and many have tried to maintain the intensive family feeling and antidrug community found in therapeutic communities (Akers, 1992).

Nonresidential Programs

The therapeutic community movement also inspired a whole array of nonresidential programs, drop-in centers, hot lines, and "rap" centers in the 1970s, designed especially for adolescents and offering peer-group talk and counseling on drug problems whether or not the youngster had serious drug abuse problems (Akers, 1992).

Residential Programs

The best-known residential programs are those that attempt to provide a "therapeutic-community" environment promoting an entirely drug-free lifestyle. The programs offer social support for a positive, nondrug dependent image of oneself, and help individuals who have reached bottom regain control of their lives (Akers, 1992). These programs may be either publicly or privately operated.

Self-Help Groups

Historically, the most popular and widely used self-help model is that of 12-step recovery programs such as Alcoholics Anonymous (AA). They can serve as a valuable source for social support, peer identification, and role modeling and offer an effective conceptual framework for relapse prevention and successful recovery (Washton, 1988). Members gain strength and security from meeting with others who understand and share their concerns and who can offer practical strategies for surviving "one day at a time" (Gold, 1992). In addition to their effectiveness when used in conjunction with a treatment program, the ongoing nature, wide availability, and absence of fees of 12-step programs support the notion that recovery is a lifelong process involving permanent changes in attitude and lifestyle (Washton, 1988). The programs are based on 12 steps that help members focus on gaining strength toward lasting recovery. By accepting and carrying out the 12 steps and attending meetings regularly, many are able to reduce their sense of isolation and demoralization, leading to a better chance for remaining abstinent (Millman, 1988). The process of recovery, especially through the 12-step program of AA, involves the development of a new sense of self, new beliefs and values, and new ways of relating to oneself and the world (Brown, 1985).

Other self-help models have been developed, although they are not widespread. Participation is voluntary and draws on patients' motivation to take greater responsibility and control of their lives.

Rational Recovery

Rational Recovery (RR) is a self-help program that distinguishes itself from the traditional 12-step programs. Associated with the

Institute for Rational-Emotive Therapy, RR stresses self-control and the power of the individual. It may appeal especially to patients who do not accept the concept of the "higher power" that is the basis of AA (Table 8–1). Rational Recovery differs from the traditional 12-step programs in its assertion that a person can recover from addiction, rather than always being in recovery (Galanter, Egelko, & Edwards, 1993). Similar programs that have been advocated include Women for Sobriety and the Secular Organization for Sobriety (SOS).

Alcoholics Anonymous

Alcoholics Anonymous is an international fellowship of men and women who once had a drinking problem. It is nonprofessional, self-supporting, nondenominational, multiracial, apolitical, and available almost everywhere. There are no age or education requirements. Membership is open to anyone who wants to do something about his or her drinking problem.

AA was founded in 1935 by New York stockbroker Bill Wilson, who created a fellowship under a cloak of strict anonymity. The "drunk," to use a popular AA word, often admits his or her alcoholism before the group, acknowledging that alcoholism is a disease for which abstinence is the only answer (Table 8–1). Most adherents also believe they will never recover but instead will always be "in recovery." Although many who feel they have been saved by AA cannot explain how or why it works, they do believe they stay sober by helping others stay sober too (Gleick, 1995).

Al-Anon

Al-Anon is a self-help fellowship based on the 12 suggested steps of Alcoholics Anonymous. Anyone who feels their life has been affected by close contact with a problem drinker is eligible for membership in Al-Anon (Al-Anon Family Group Headquarters, Inc., 1987).

Alateen

Alateen is a fellowship of teenage relatives and friend of alcoholics. Alateen is a part of Al-Anon. Young people meet to help each other cope with the troubles brought about by another person's drinking. Alateen is not for teenage alcoholics or drug

Table 8-1. The 12 Steps of Alcoholics Anonymous.

1. We admitted we were powerless over alcohol—that our lives had become unmanageable.
2. Came to believe that a Power greater than ourselves could restore us to sanity.
3. Made a decision to turn our will and our lives to the care of God, *as we understood Him.*
4. Made a searching and fearless moral inventory.
5. Admitted to God, to ourselves and to another human being the exact nature of our wrongs.
6. Were entirely ready to have God remove all these defects of character.
7. Humbly asked Him to remove our shortcomings.
8. Made a list of all persons we had harmed, and became willing to make amends to them all.
9. Made direct amends to such people wherever possible, except when to do so would injure them or others.
10. Continued to take personal inventory and when we were wrong promptly admit it.
11. Sought through prayer and meditation to improve our conscious contact with God, *as we understood Him,* praying only for knowledge of His will for use and the power to carry that out.
12. Having had a spiritual awakening as the result of these steps, we tried to carry this message to alcoholics and to practice these principles in all our affairs.

Source: The Twelve Steps are reprinted with permission of Alcoholics Anonymous World Services, Inc. Permission to reprint the Twelve Steps does not mean that AA has reviewed or approved the contents of this publication, nor that AA agrees with the views expressed herein. AA is a program of recovery from alcoholism *only*—use of the Twelve Steps in connection with programs and activities which are patterned after AA, but which address other problems, or in any other non-AA context, does not imply otherwise.

abusers unless their lives have been affected by someone else's drinking (Al-Anon Family Group Headquarters, Inc., 1991).

Outpatient Treatment

Intensive outpatient programs were modeled after psychiatric day treatment programs, which emerged in the 1970s as alternatives to inpatient hospitalizations. They vary considerably in the amount of time that patients are treated. General outpatient services are used as primary treatment or as extended aftercare following completion of an inpatient or intensive outpatient program. These types of services usually include weekly group therapy sessions with an alcoholism counselor, participation in AA meetings, and family therapy when appropriate (Bradley, 1992; Ellis & McClure, 1992; Institute of Medicine, 1990a).

Chemical Dependency Programs

Chemical dependency (CD) programs generally are residential or inpatient, with a 3- to 6-week duration, followed by up to 2 years of attending self-help groups or a weekly outpatient therapy group. CD programs are based on an AA (12-step) idea of personal change and the belief that vulnerability to dependence is a permanent but controllable disability. The goals of CD programs are those of total abstinence and lifestyle alteration (Institute of Medicine, 1990b).

RELAPSE PREVENTION STRATEGIES

Relapse during the recovery process can be triggered by a variety of factors. These include stress, depression, and levels of alcohol craving and withdrawal, negative life events and daily inconveniences that an individual experiences, as well as interpersonal tension. Relapse prevention strategies have been developed to teach alcoholics how to cope effectively with potential relapse triggers.

Common Symptoms Leading to Possible Relapse

- Exhaustion
- Impatience
- Depression
- Self-pity
- "It Can't Happen to Me"
- Expecting Too Much
- Letting Up on Disciplines
- Forgetting Gratitude
- Dishonesty
- Argumentativeness
- Frustration
- Cockiness
- Use of Chemicals
- Wanting Too Much
- Complacency

Relapse Prevention

Craving and urges are normal for a patient who is attempting to abstain from alcohol (Kadden et al., 1992). It is helpful to devise other methods for coping with cravings before they occur. Some strategies may include: becoming involved with a distracting activity such as exercising or going to a movie; talking through the craving with a friend or member of a self-help group; challenging and changing one's thoughts by keeping a list of the negative consequences of abuse and the positive reasons for being abstinent; and urge surfing.

Urge Surfing

Urge surfing is a technique that likens urges to ocean waves; that is, they are small when they start, will grow in size, and then will break up and dissipate. Urge surfing is composed of three basic steps: (1) taking an inventory of the craving experience as it affects the body; (2) focusing on one area where the urge is being felt and noticing what is occurring; and (3) repeating the focusing process with each part of the body that experiences the craving. The purpose of urge surfing is to experience the cravings in a new way and to *ride them out* until they go away (Kadden et al., 1992).

Training is designed to increase the patient's ability to avoid or cope with high-risk situations and to reduce the probability of relapse (Marlatt & Gordon, 1985). It seeks to teach patients strategies for avoiding high-risk situations; strategies for coping with high-risk situations when encountered; strategies for coping with cravings; and strategies for coping with lapses in alcohol use to prevent full-blown relapses. Classical relapse prevention approaches make a distinction between "slips" and relapses, with slips defined as mild episodes of use that are viewed as learning experiences.

Assisting Patients in Developing Relapse Prevention Skills

The following may assist the patient in the development of relapse prevention skills:

(continued)

(continued)

- Developing new coping skills for handling high-risk situations
- Making lifestyle changes to decrease the need for alcohol
- Increasing participation in health activities
- Understanding relapse as a process and an event
- Understanding and dealing with social pressures to drink
- Developing a supportive relapse prevention network
- Developing methods of coping with negative emotional states
- Learning methods of coping with cognitive distortions
- Developing a plan to interrupt a slip or relapse
- Recognizing the warning signs of relapse
- Combating powerful memories of euphoria
- Reinforcing negative aspects of alcohol
- Overcoming the desire to regain control over drinking
- Avoiding people, places, and things that may trigger urges
- Developing an array of pleasurable and rewarding alternatives (Kleber, 1994, p. 35)

Relapse can have two possible impacts on the person. It can confront the individual with the undeniable reality of his or her illness and the need to pursue treatment. In this case, relapse can be termed "therapeutic," meaning the end consequence is progress toward accepting and constructively dealing with the illness. The second impact can be to reinforce mistaken attitudes about the disease and about life. When this happens, a recurring relapse pattern will develop. Relapse, therefore can generate either positive or negative consequences in terms of future improvements in life situations.

SUMMARY

As with all treatments in medicine and surgery, not all treatment works for all patients. Rather, a treatment should be selected based on the needs of the specific patient. Also, combinations of treatments are often necessary.

The total course of dependence can be influenced by adequate treatment for which health care providers have a direct responsibility. Regardless of any treatment difficulties, providers must continue to apply all knowledge available in an attempt to eliminate the syndrome of alcohol dependence and treat any associated psychopathology (Council on Mental Health, 1971).

CHAPTER 9

NEW AGE TREATMENTS

- The Mind-Body Connection
- Techniques

Most people who try unconventional therapies are simply seeking other options (Table 9–1), many believing that these new natural health remedies offer them the opportunity to take some control of the management of their health. The main thesis of alternative medicine is that it promotes wellness. Physicians argue in rebuttal that many of the optimistic claims, for example, improved resistance to disease, heightened fitness, and enhanced longevity are based on faith, optimism, and little more. Scientific proof of efficacy is conspicuously lacking or inconclusive in supporting the health benefit of most categories of alternative treatment and remedy.

THE MIND-BODY CONNECTION

Mind and body are not separate phenomena, they are both aspects of one information system. Life is an information system. Biology is a process of information transduction. Mind and body are two facets or two ways of conceptualizing this single infor-

Table 9–1. New Age Treatments.

Cutaneous Stimulation	*Distraction*
Massage	Visual concentration
Pain relief with heat, cold, or both	Slow rhythmic breathing
Ice application or massage for pain relief	Sing and tap rhythm
Active listening to music	Laughter
	Describing a series of pictures
Relaxation	***Imagery***
Deep rhythmic breathing	Hypnosis and imagery
Humor for relaxation	Emptying the sandbox
Centering exercises	Breathing out pain
Jaw relaxation	Ball of healing energy
Peaceful past experiences	
Meditation	
Progressive relaxation	
Yoga	
Simple touch, massage, or warmth for relaxation	
Biofeedback techniques	
Acupuncture	
Acupressure	
Desensitization of stressful moments	

mation system. Medical science has specialized in all the anatomical, physiological, and pharmacological methods of accessing and facilitating healing; it has focused almost exclusively on the "body side" of the mind-body equation. In this section, alternative techniques based on the utilization of psychological factors are explored. The majority of these techniques may be learned and practiced by the alcohol-dependent physically challenged patient, either in a rehabilitation or home setting.

TECHNIQUES

Acupuncture

Professionals are beginning to consider acupuncture in treatment for alcohol and drug addiction. Acupuncture—the use of thin needles inserted subcutaneously into the body at specific points that represent centers of energy (Katims, Ng, & Lowinson, 1992)—may provide some symptom relief for patients having difficulty managing anxiety, or it may be used as an adjunct to outpatient detoxification from alcohol (Alling, Johnson, & Elmoghazy, 1990; Ter Reit, Kleijnen, & Knipschild, 1990; Whitehead, 1978).

For centuries, acupuncture has been used in Far Eastern countries as a therapy for a variety of ailments. It is believed that the normal functioning of the body depends on a balance of two opposite polar energies, yin and yang. These energies flow along lines of the body called meridians. There are approximately 1,000 acupuncture points along each meridian. Stimulation of the points by needles is believed to correct the imbalance of energy flow, release blockages of energy, and enhance the body's natural capacity to heal itself (Nebelkopf, 1981; Wen & Cheung, 1973).

Acupuncture may be most helpful as an adjunct to other therapies (Crowe & Reeves, 1994) for patients who seek outpatient, nonpharmacological treatment alternatives for alcohol dependence (Bullock, Culliton, & Olander 1989; Smith, 1986).

Biofeedback

Biofeedback uses technology to help patients learn relaxation. The foundation of biofeedback is the premise that, if patients can develop a sensory awareness of an involuntary function, they can learn to change it. For example, in a biofeedback setup, temperature sensors are connected to patients' fingers, and skin temperature is converted to an audible signal. The faster the beeps, the higher the temperature. The patients raise their body temperatures, consequently increasing the tones. Body temperature is a measure of blood flow, which is regulated by the autonomic nervous system. In order to raise skin temperature the patients must relax their sympathetic nervous systems (Weil, 1990). When the patients relax the correct area, positive reinforcement is provided by the tones, assisting them to enhance their skill.

There are many applications for biofeedback. It may be utilized to decrease muscle tension, for pain control, and so forth. Once learned, the patient should spend 15 to 20 minutes a day practicing the technique.

Relaxation Techniques to Reduce Internal Stress

A healthy diet and a program of regular exercise are the two best stress reducers available. Others include deep rhythmic breathing, acupuncture, biofeedback, acupressure and other types of massage, yoga, progressive relaxation technique, desensitization of stressful moments, and meditation techniques.

In identifying stress, you may want to consider administering the STRESS AUDIT, a self-administered questionnaire that assists patients in identifying areas of their lives that are stressful, their stress symptoms, and their vulnerability to stress. The relationship between stress and physical and/or emotional symptoms is discussed with the patients, raising their level of awareness regarding the impact of external and internal stimuli on stress (Weil, 1990).

Breathing

When an individual is anxious, breathing becomes quick and shallow, originating from the top of the chest. The most effective relaxation technique is the conscious regulation of breathing. Health care professionals can teach patients how to breathe properly with the following exercise, and tell them to practice it for 2 to 5 minutes at least once daily and whenever they are feeling anxious (Weil, 1990).

Instruct the patient to sit up straight and to place the left hand on the stomach, and the right hand on the chest. Next, instruct the patient to inhale slowly. Ask the patient to visualize the lungs filling up with air from the bottom up, so that the left hand rises before their right hand does. Then, instruct the patient to exhale slowly and steadily, top to bottom, reversing the process.

Progressive Relaxation

Progressive relaxation is a way of releasing tension in muscles. There are many variations. Most begin by having individuals lie on their backs in a comfortable position. Instruct the patients to take a series of deep slow breaths and then focus their awareness on different parts of their bodies, becoming aware of any muscular tension and releasing it. One way to do this is to instruct patients to tense a muscle deliberately and then relax it. Following this, instruct the patients to lie still with their eyes closed, concentrating on their breathing (Weil, 1990).

Exercise

When appropriate, exercise can be recommended to the patient. It can be relaxing and a great way to reduce stress. For example, if individuals are experiencing feelings of anger or frustration, a brisk walk will often put them back in a good mood (Weil, 1990). After 20 minutes of continuous activity, the body begins to produce endorphins—biochemicals that act as natural tranquilizers.

Some patients report that regular exercise reduces cravings and seems to level out their moods. Its efficacy may be secondary to it being a specific nonalcohol-related activity that affects feelings.

Yoga

Yoga is an excellent promotor of relaxation. It is not a religion; it is one of the most practical systems of personal development in the world (Stahl, 1992).

There are four main paths of yoga. The one that is the focus of this section is Raja yoga, the science of physical and mental control. The subdivision of Raja known as Hatha yoga emphasizes posture and breath regulation.

Yoga, although one of the oldest and most holistic systems of mind-body fitness, is totally relevant to contemporary life. Literally translated, yoga means union, and it aims to attain unity of consciousness—mind, body, and spiritual health. It induces spiritual awareness, deep relaxation, mental tranquillity, concentration, and clarity, fused with physical strength (Krista, 1986). Yoga encourages a positive attitude toward self-acceptance, self-nurturing, and self-mastery, which are important elements in functioning as a well balanced adult.

The physical aspect of Raja yoga, known as Hatha yoga, includes a number of *asanas* or poses. Yoga asanas are performed slowly and meditatively, combined with deep abdominal breathing. These movements awaken awareness and restore control of the body, as well as have an effect spiritually—freeing the individual from fears and helping to instill confidence and serenity (Weil, 1990).

Massage and Body Work

There is a great deal of evidence that the state of mind and nervous system is reflected in the state of the musculature, and also that body work is one route into the unconsciousness mind (Weil, 1990). Massage is more a symptomatic treatment than a lasting change. It is also limited in its application.

Visualization and Guided Imagery

Visualization and guided imagery work with the connection between the visual brain and the involuntary nervous system. When this portion of the brain (the visual cortex at the back of the head) is not occupied with input from the eyes, it seems to be able to influence physical and emotional states. You can learn this technique from books, from self-help tapes, or from instructors.

The best times for practice are the transition states between sleeping and waking, just before falling asleep or just after waking. At these times it passes more easily into your unconscious mind, allowing for relaxation of the body and nervous system.

Centering Exercise

Find a comfortable position and close your eyes. First notice your breathing. Do not try to change it but merely notice how you are breathing now. Where does your breath go? How deep is it? Does it stop at your chest? Does it fill your stomach? What is your rate of breathing? Are you breathing fast or slow? Ask yourself, is this the way I normally breath?

Now, as you are paying attention, consciously make the choice to deepen your breathing. Pull the air in so that your chest fills and your stomach fills and rises like a balloon. Then let the air out slowly and fully. Pull the air in with the same steady, slow pace. As you breathe in think to yourself, "IN" and "OUT." Breathe in the air and then release it finding a natural rhythm of your own.

Now maintain your deep breathing but turn your attention to the rest of your body. Starting with your scalp and forehead, move down your body looking for places of tightness or tension or pain. If you find a place that feels tight, tighten that place even tighter, as tight as you can, and then release. Move to your facial muscles, the back of your neck, and your throat, and each time you find a tightness or tension, a place where the anger or frustration or fatigue of the day is locked, tighten that place as tight as you can, and then release.

Check your shoulders, your arms, your hands, and your fingers. Move to your chest, your spine, and your lower back, tighten and release at each spot of tension. Check your abdomen and your genitals, your thighs, knees, calves. Finally check your ankles, your feet, your toes.

Each part of your body is feeling heavier now; more relaxed; more in touch with you and your inner self. And finally let the inner self take the last stray thoughts and concerns from the day and imagine a lovely glass jar. A jar with a lid. That jar can be any size or shape and color you want. Put those thoughts and worries in your jar and put the cap on it. Put the jar away on a shelf. You can go back and find those thoughts and concerns later if you need them, but for right now you are ready to turn yourself and your attention to other things, including the people and events that will make up the rest of the day/evening. You will be focused so you can be fully here and fully your inner self. Allow that focus to turn on this room. Imagine the room as it was when you closed your eyes, and when you are ready, open and rejoin us.

Meditation

Meditation is directed concentration. Meditators learn to focus their awareness and direct it on an object. The relaxation response has been shown to produce a healthy reduction in blood pressure, decreases in heart and respiratory rates, and an increase in blood flow. Some use it to soothe chronic pain and physicians teach it to treat insomnia and to overcome infertility when the cause is stress (Williams, 1996).

Meditation can be learned in a number of ways: through books, instructional tapes, meditation classes, or meditation retreats. It can be done in any position, but most recommend a seated posture with the spine straight. Meditation should be done every day without fail, with 20 to 30 minutes as a reasonable length of time.

Mantram

Mantram is the practice of repeating over and over in the mind certain syllables, words, or phrases that help unify consciousness and counteract negative mental states. Repetition of a verbal formula is a way of focusing the mind and counteracting the damage done to both mind and body by thoughts that produce anxiety, agitation, and unhappiness. Repetition of a mantram provides a comforting focus for the mind. It is a totally portable technique, requires no training or equipment, and can be used in any circumstance. Mantrams are especially helpful for people with restless minds, whose turbulent thoughts keep them from relaxing, concentrating, and falling asleep.

Hypnotherapy

Hypnotherapy, also referred to as hypnosis, is accepted as a useful method for relaxation, pain control, and management of habits like smoking and overeating. In fact, the use of trance and suggestion to affect the unconscious mind and the regulatory systems of the body has many more potential applications in the treatment of disease.

Hypnotherapists do not put an individual into a trance; they arrange circumstances to increase the likelihood of having the patient shift into a trance state, which is part of the normal repertory of human consciousness.

Expressive Art Therapy

Artistic expression, including journal writing, can play a vital role in treatment. It often serves as a useful adjunct to physical and psychotherapies.

Recreational Therapy

Recreational therapy, which has played an active role in physical rehabilitation programs, can also be beneficial in the treatment of the alcohol-dependent patient. Recreational therapists can help patients overcome denial and help change behavior.

One particularly effective strategy in recreational therapy is the use of "new games" used in conjunction with the 12 Steps of Alcoholics Anonymous. The patients may become so involved in the game or activity that they are not consciously aware of their own behaviors, helping both patients and therapist identify unconscious patterns in normal life. Asking patients to try to juggle some recreational equipment, for example, may lead to insight as to how they balance their problems. If what the patients say conflicts with the behavior shown in the activity, the therapist can confront the conflict, moving the patients through struggles like denial. It becomes much more difficult for people to deny their behaviors when reacting in a certain manner without consciously thinking.

Herbal Therapy

Herbal therapy enhances the quality of life by strengthening the body in places where it is needed. Many herbs contain vitamins and minerals that provide nourishment and support to the body. For example, the dandelion leaf provides vitamin A and nettle contains iron and calcium.

Herbal therapy is individualized based on what a person's body needs assistance with. For example, if an individual is having chemotherapy, an herbalist would recommend he or she use an herb that would provide nourishment and support to the immune system. The use of herbs is one more piece to the wellness pie.

Sleep Disturbances

Sleep disturbance is a common feature of withdrawal, anxiety, and depression. The following suggestions can be offered to patients who either anticipate difficulty or are having difficulty with insomnia: (1) Go to bed at the same time every night and get up at a regular time, no matter how little sleep you actually get. (2) Do not nap. (3) Do not consume caffeine after 6:00 P.M. Also avoid cigarette smoking at night, because nicotine is a stimulant. (4) Engage in regular exercise if appropriate, preferably at the same time of day, as exercise appears to help normalize sleep patterns. (5) Calcium and el-tryptophan (both of which are found in milk) are nature's pacifiers and may calm and relax the patient (Zweben & O'Connell, 1992).

Other psychological strategies, such as the use of relaxation tapes or exercises, playing soft music, or deep breathing or centering exercises may be employed. Some patients need to be reminded to avoid initiating a difficult discussion with their spouse or children before bedtime, and to reduce stimulation in general. Although these recommendations may take several days to a week to help, they do tend to be effective if the patient is able to maintain them (Zweben & O'Connell, 1992).

SUMMARY

Clearly, the more techniques health care professionals can offer to help their patients throughout the rehabilitation process, the more likely they are to succeed with those patients. In addition, what works for some patients may not work for others. That is why it makes sense to offer a broad range of rehabilitation techniques.

CHAPTER 10

REHABILITATION OF THE ALCOHOL-DEPENDENT DISABLED PATIENT

- **Disability and the Family**
- **The Continuum of Care**
- **The Rehabilitation Process**
- **Aftercare**

Severe disorders of the mind or brain, perhaps to a greater degree than any other single area of health care, lead to complex interactions of medical, social, and often legal issues. That is, problems are created which refuse to be confined to any one sphere. Just as a patient may be referred among specialists, these problems demand simultaneous attention of both medical (here, meaning biomedical or biological) and nonmedical aspects.

The nature and extent of alcohol dependency not only plays a critical role in the causation of many kinds of functional deficits in the neurologically/medically impaired, but also may preclude remediation or resolution of these deficits (Heinemann, Doll, & Schnoll, 1989). Alcoholism is as difficult for all caregivers involved with the patient, to deal with, as it is crippling for the patient. Moreover, the behavioral alterations that a patient may experience as a result of alcohol abuse may require specific modifications in the design of rehabilitative treatments and/or in the formulation of attainable goals.

Rehabilitation aids patients in moving from dependence to independence as they gain optimal function. In working toward this goal, increasing patient involvement is the key, while the health care professional is the catalyst. Thus, rehabilitation stresses patient and family participation and cooperation throughout the recovery process.

DISABILITY AND THE FAMILY

The diagnosis of a disability can evoke negative reactions—shock, denial, anger, depression, resentment, guilt, and embarrassment (Shaw & McMahon, 1990), impacting every family member. Unfortunately, this emotional process of adjustment is compounded when the disabled individual is also abusing alcohol. In fact, the emotional reactions to alcohol abuse can be similar to those involving a disability.

The presence of a person with a disability who is also involved in alcohol abuse or the presence of two family members, one with a disability and the other involved in alcohol abuse, hits the family hard. The stress created by the presence of a disability is significant. Adding alcohol abuse to it geometrically increases the stress on a family. The stresses intertwine. The coping and corrective strategies become so complex as to be overwhelming.

Very often, the alcohol abuse is pre-existing and the family has adjusted to living with the alcoholic. However, in the case of a newly acquired disability, alcohol abuse may go unrecognized because the family is focusing on disability to the exclusion of all other concerns. Sometimes symptoms are missed because disability-related problems can be similar to those generated through alcohol abuse. For example, family members may believe that medical problems, such as bed sores or recurring infections, are due strictly to a disability, when the reason may be continued misuse of alcohol. As with families living with alcoholics, even if the cause is recognized, they may be unable or unwilling to explore some of the difficult actions necessary to address the problem.

It can be very difficult to practice "letting go" and "tough love" on a family member who is disabled. The emotional impact is exacerbated by a lack of objectivity. As family members and significant others become involved in the rehabilitation process, the following guidelines can be beneficial in assisting the entire family to deal with alcohol misuse and disability.

- Family members can become educated about alcohol and its relationship to disabilities. You may suggest readings, attending training sessions, talking to counselors or health educators, or attending self-help groups (such as Al-Anon or AA).
- Families should encourage participation in peer groups or support groups. The disabled family member should be provided opportunities to make his or her own decisions. And the family should be instructed that they can be supportive by giving the person with the disability the right to learn from his or her own mistakes.
- If family members are concerned about the alcohol use of the person with a disability, these concerns should be expressed in a caring but firm way. Boundaries and logical consequences should be set regarding alcohol use. The consequences should be stated in advance, be enforceable, and age-appropriate.
- Families dealing with either alcohol abuse or disability, or both, should seek professional assistance when needed. Either of these conditions can dramatically alter family interactions, causing alienation and breakdowns in the family unit.

THE CONTINUUM OF CARE

Every patient is an individual with inherent rights. Perhaps the most important of these is the right to whatever assistance is necessary to achieve full potential in every aspect of recovery. This approach is holistic for alcoholism affects the total patient and his or her family. The physical, psychological, emotional, vocational, educational, civic, spiritual, and financial effects all must be taken into consideration.

As a health care provider in a rehabilitation setting, you play a central role in the rehabilitation process, both as an advocate for the patient and as a coordinator and provider of care. You are responsible for assessing the patient's needs; developing a plan in consultation with the patient, family, and other health care professionals; and monitoring the patient's progress throughout the rehabilitation continuum. You are also concerned with many areas of the patient's care that may influence the rehabilitation process. These include frustration, feelings of powerlessness, depression, infection or sepsis, complications of decreased mobility (i.e., skin breakdown, venous status, renal calculi), potential for self-harm, noncompliance, and dependence in activities of daily living.

The rehabilitative process follows a continuum, from admission to return to home and community as a productive citizen. The patient's physical and mental capabilities must be assessed carefully throughout this process. After the process of alcohol detoxification has been completed, alcohol-free treatment can begin emphasizing the development of new coping skills that are essential for an alcohol-free life (NIH, 1993).

Throughout rehabilitation, the emphasis should be on the patients' abilities, striving to convert the patients' "do for me" attitude to a "help me do for myself" attitude. Whenever possible, work in terms of the patients' priorities and concerns, and encourage them to participate in their care. This involvement allows patients some control over their lives and bodies, and is essential for self-esteem. Limit the choices to simple tasks patients will be able to perform successfully. Let patients determine which tasks are most important to them. Again, making choices encourages patients to assume independence.

Making contracts with patients is a useful way of motivating them to meet their goals. By contracting, the patient "owns" the goal and the patient knows in advance exactly what is expected and when. As the patient becomes more involved in rehabilitation, the emphasis shifts increasingly to independence.

Adjustment to Permanent Disability

Persons who sustain disabling injuries have psychological reactions that make it difficult to establish positive relationships. These individuals are faced with many losses: the use of limbs and body functions, an accustomed lifestyle, self-esteem and identity, values and independence, the ability to work, and friends or spouse, who may be unable to cope.

These patients will grieve over their losses. In caring for them, understanding their grief is crucial to lessening their anxiety and frustration. Patients may go four stages before finally adapting to their losses.

Anger and Denial. During this stage, patients focus their emotions inward. Health care providers may become the objects of hostility, anger, and rage, and patients may resist all social contact.

Denial that anything is wrong may be evident, and may reflect the patient's attempt to maintain his or her preinjury status. It may also be an attempt to cope with drastic changes in lifestyle: patterns of relating, self-image, independence, and autonomy.

Defensive Retreat. Acknowledging their injury, but still unable to accept the possibility of permanent disability, patients defend themselves by retreating into a fantasy of full recovery.

Acknowledgment. Reality now sets in and patients may become greatly distressed, recognizing the extent and severity of their injury. Patients' value systems may be shaken, especially if health, physical activity, independence, mobility, and self-support were of particular importance. It is during this stage that patients' despair may lead them to suicide.

Adaptation. At this stage, patients begin to plan attainable goals. They begin to cope with their disabilities and realize that other things can be accomplished. Focus shifts from the past to the future.

Dealing with Resistance

Resistance to therapy can be diffused if health care providers recognize their own role in it and change the way it is addressed. Resistance is often confused with denial because both terms can define similar processes. The resistance referred to here is emotional physics in which patients may not deny that there is a problem—physical or alcohol—but find that their belief system impedes change.

An accurate and helpful approach to resistance lies in acknowledging that resistance is a process that is indigenous to the therapeutic relationship and not necessarily a problem that the patient has. The presence of resistance may indicate that the patient is actually moving toward health and is an indication of tension leading to the next phase of wellness.

Mutual Respect

Absolutely vital to successful treatment is the nature of the interpersonal relationship that develops between the caregiver and the patient. Winning the trust, confidence, and respect of the patient constitutes the first major task to be accomplished. This cannot be achieved unless the health care providers involved adhere strictly to the tenets of confidentiality. Even implied threats of reporting, except under extreme emergency conditions, may completely destroy the basis required for continuing therapy (Council on Mental Health, 1971).

Health care providers must show an active interest in the patient and his or her struggles. They must identify and acknowledge positive aspects of the patient's personality and behavior, so that the patient does not feel that the health care provider is just another critical member of the establishment. Alcohol-dependent persons have been lectured to and scolded, often for years, by parents, spouses, friends, employers, and probation officers; they are hypersensitive to criticism, which has come to signify rejection. Careful choice of words is required in establishing communication and in avoiding an implication of condescension or hostility (Council on Mental Health, 1971).

The alcohol-dependent disabled patient's denial system seems to cause the greatest difficulty for health care providers. For example, denial is said to be present in most alcoholics. Many professionals focus on confronting patients' denials about their drinking (Mourer, 1992). However, to focus on denial in regard to drinking in patients with a newly acquired spinal cord injury may disturb their capacity to appropriately modulate information about their injury. Professionals must remember that patients are also coping with the uncertainty related to their loss of functioning. In many cases, denial is an important aspect of the patient adaptation and adjustment to the new injury. Professionals must assess the patients' ability to process and understand the information being provided to them, and provide patients with the opportunity to work through each adjustment phase at their own pace (Mourer, 1992).

It is hard to see these patients as capable of making their lives satisfying when confronted with their profound distortion of reality. Instead of breaking a person's denial, nurture his or her accurate insight, communicating a much more respectful message. You must still confront the discrepancies in a patient's thoughts and behavior as well as provide education about alcoholism, recovery, and disabilities. Remember, however, that patients have a right to deal with their disease in their own way. Do not operate from an expectation that the patients will, should, or must deal with the addiction or the disability.

Enabling the Disabled

Individuals with disabilities who abuse alcohol rarely manage to hide this fact completely. However, in spite of the sometimes obvious symptoms, others may not recognize or react to abuse when it affects someone with a disability. This is referred to as enabling. Because of inappropriate reactions to disabilities, enabling of alcohol abuse can be particularly problematic for the disabled individual.

Ironically, in the terminology of disability advocacy, to enable someone with a disability means to provide physically and attitudinally flexible environments that maximize societal participation. There needs to be a balance between being flexible and understanding about disability-related limitations, without encouraging alcohol use. Finding this balance is challenging for those who are dealing with the issue of alcohol abuse and disability.

Overcompensation by well-meaning family members, friends, or professionals actually can increase attention on the disability, rather than on other attributes of the person. When this occurs, alcohol abuse symptoms are more likely to be perceived as disability-related. Even when the abuse is recognized, there is a tendency to accept that the disability makes the abuse more understandable. Often those closest to the abuser are the least able to recognize their own enabling behaviors.

On some occasions, societal reactions include a more active form of alcohol abuse enabling. Individuals may feel that life with a disability is so unpleasant that there is an "entitlement" to use alcohol in order to cope (Moore, 1990; Moore & Ford, 1991). This mistaken belief encourages persons with disabilities to utilize alcohol and other drugs without facing the societal constraints applied to the general population.

The enabling of alcohol abuse among those with disabilities can best be addressed through education and self-evaluation. Appropriate responses to alcohol abuse and disability issues require that a person be comfortable with his or her own relationship with alcohol. If there are personal issues of alcohol abuse or codependency, it may be more difficult to respond to these symptoms in others. Also, a person must be comfortable interacting with a disabled person. If there is discomfort related to being around someone with a disability, it is likely that alcohol abuse issues will ignored completely.

The same criteria for reacting to alcohol abuse should be used for everyone, regardless of whether or not they are disabled. The task facing rehabilitation professionals includes educating people with disabilities and others about the dangers inherent in alcohol use. Family members of a disabled person must learn to accept the disability with sensitivity, while acknowledging the accompanying risks for alcohol abuse.

THE REHABILITATION PROCESS

Alcohol use and dependence typically make it difficult for patients to participate in the rehabilitation process. Some preliminary studies of trauma patients have shown that these patients experience a more complicated medical course of inpatient treatment and longer hospitalizations (Mishkin & Sparadeo, 1991; Sparadeo & Gill, 1989).

Once the patient's limitations have been identified, rehabilitation efforts can then be directed toward working with caretakers who are responsible for the patient and engineering living arrangements to make the most of the patient's residual capacities. The realistic appraisal of treatment goals requires identification of several key elements: a clear neurological/medical diagnosis; an understanding of the specific natural history and course of recovery from the disease; the secondary medical complications that may constrain recovery; the specific makeup of the patient's existing functional deficits; the precise nature of the patient's underlying neuropsychological functioning; and pre-existing environmental or lifestyle factors that may preclude systematic psychosocial change. Only after consideration of these contributors to a patient's behavior can the best treatment regimes in relation to the rehabilitation goals be established.

Treatment Approaches

The patient with multiple disabilities challenges health care providers in numerous ways. Until recently, patients with brain injuries, speech handicaps, mental disabilities, hearing problems, or comprehension incapacity were unable to benefit from the usual group educational and individual counseling modalities of alcoholism treatment. However, what most professionals will find is that the conventional treatment options so often available for alcohol-dependent individuals may not be able to meet the specific needs of the alcohol-dependent individual who is disabled. There is increasing recognition of the need for integrated programs for disabled patients that address the patients' physical, cognitive, motor, and personality deficits. In most cases, specific treatment plans and linkages with specific community agencies will need to be initiated prior to hospital discharge.

One of the issues facing professionals caring for patients with disabilities is the rationalizations often offered by these patients. They may rationalize that their disabling injury will lead them to end their chronic drinking. To effectively respond to these patients, health care professionals must have full understanding of the relationship between alcohol abuse and disabilities (Schmelzer, 1994).

For some disabled patients, any use of alcohol can be very dangerous. Even small amounts can have very negative effects, possibly causing seizures or problems with circulation. It is imperative that patients, their families, friends, and significant others be educated regarding the effects of alcohol. For example, alcohol can produce a dangerous reaction if taken with certain antibiotics. Symptoms include headache, rapid pulse, increased respiration, and vomiting. Alcohol combined with other drugs can affect memory and problem-solving ability, decrease reaction time, interfere with prescribed relaxants, and may even cause fatal reactions.

Setting Appropriate Goals

It is important to discuss the effects of alcohol on rehabilitative functions. For example, it is probably wasteful and even unkind to enter a patient with late stages of Wernicke-Korsakoff syndrome in a rehabilitation training program to improve cognitive function when the disease has rendered that patient incapable of meeting the day-to-day requirements of independently remembering, maintaining, and monitoring their ongoing responses. In proposing to improve "memory" through cognitive retraining techniques, well-intentioned rehabilitation specialists have overlooked that they are placing the patient in an inherent paradox: if learning is impaired, then learning to learn will also be impaired.

Traumatic Brain Injury (TBI)

As you may recall, alcohol abuse is associated with over half of all TBIs and appears to be related to lifestyles where alcohol abuse and risk taking were common (Sparadeo, Strauss, & Barth, 1990). Survivors may seek to demonstrate their full recovery by returning to preinjury levels of alcohol use or may pursue a preinjury "comfort level" of intoxication to prevent unwanted withdrawal symptoms (Sparadeo & Gill, 1989).

Some brain injuries are associated with decreases in certain brain chemicals and a patient's use of alcohol may be an attempt to compensate for this deficiency. However, because of the brain injury, these patients may experience stronger effects from smaller amounts of alcohol than prior to the injury. Resumption of alcohol use may significantly exacerbate cognitive deficits, cause worsening of memory functioning, and place the patient at a high risk for reinjury.

Specialized alcohol abuse treatment often is necessary for people with traumatic brain injury. TBI can include lasting memory and cognitive difficulties, and alcohol treatment needs should be addressed by taking learning styles and capacities into consideration.

Prevention of relapse to alcohol abuse might be best approached by emphasizing the effects of alcohol on the damaged brain and the person's recovery from TBI. Following are some points that may be emphasized in a discussion with a person with TBI (Langley, 1991):

- The disinhibiting effects of alcohol are not helpful when disinhibition itself is a social problem for many patients with TBI.
- The depressant effects of alcohol are not helpful when proneness to major reactive depressive episodes is common among people recovering from TBI.
- The effects of alcohol may interfere with medications designed to prevent seizures. They also may lower the seizure threshold.
- It is highly undesirable to exacerbate deficits in planning, verbal fluency, motor control, concentration, attention, memory, and information processing, that may already exist in the person recovering from TBI.

Working with patients recovering from TBI can become frustrating for health care professionals. It is important to remember that success needs to be measured in small increments with this population. There are many difficulties that the patient, the family, and the health care provider may be faced with during the course of rehabilitation. Often, people with TBI may digress or change course during a conversation. Redirect them using appropriate cues and reinforcers. When teaching new skills to persons with TBI, teach them in more than one setting to maximize generalization and focus on a specific goal during each session. Never assume understanding or memory from a previous session. Always repeat the purpose, duration, and guidelines for each session. Summarize previous progress and then restate where the previous session left off. Educational material should be presented in the most effective cognitive and sensory mode. All interventions should be directive in nature, short term, goal directed, and behaviorally anchored. Accentuate positive gains using frequent social praise.

It must be understood that, because the consequences of TBI are so psychologically overwhelming, most persons experience pervasive denial. This is perfectly normal. The timing and method of confrontation about deficits, including alcohol problems, should be carefully coordinated with the rehabilitation team.

When caring for this population it is important to remember that there is a period of spontaneous neurological recovery of approximately 2 years in which significant improvements can occur. These can be sometimes augmented by extensive rehabilitation methods. Some individuals with severe TBI will eventually live independently and work competitively with supports, but rarely at the level of preinjury functioning.

Spinal Cord Injuries (SCI)

For those who work with spinal cord injury (SCI) patients, the clinical issue of substance abuse and dependence is frequently an important aspect of the clinical picture. Approximately one half or more of all SCIs occur following alcohol or drug consumption (Heinemann et al., 1989). These patients continue to be at high risk for alcohol problems after the injury (Heinemann, Keen, Donohue, & Schnoll, 1988; Sparadeo & Gill, 1989). No well-defined approaches to treatment exist for patients with spinal cord injuries. The professional must develop techniques that are very specific to the needs of the SCI patient.

Education regarding the impact of alcohol is one approach in working with SCI patients. The following points might be emphasized in a discussion with a person with SCI:

- Lowered body weight means that blood alcohol will increase more rapidly than it did before.
- Combining alcohol with daily prescribed medications increases the potential for complications (Moore & Siegel, 1989) such as impaired muscular coordination and judgment. It may increase the metabolism of the drug so that its effects are of shorter duration, or it may decrease the metabolism of the drug, resulting in a need to skip or decrease a dose. It can also increase drowsiness.
- Alcohol combined with some antibiotics can cause an alcohol-intolerance reaction.
- Alcohol consumption can adversely affect the kidneys in that it acts as a diuretic and causes excessive water loss. It can cause a urinary tract infection, urinary incontinence by interrupting a catheterization schedule, or cause spontaneous voiding.

Many SCI patients drive, and the risk of reinjury from alcohol use is ever-present. More often than not, these patients are prescribed antispasmodic medications that may interact with alcohol, producing additional impairment. Although patients with spinal cord injuries may have experienced severe loss in terms of paralysis, reinjury could involve head trauma, resulting in additional loss. In light of these considerations, the use of alcohol is contraindicated in patients with spinal cord injuries.

It is especially important that members of the rehabilitation team and the patient create treatment strategies and approaches in a cooperative and collaborative manner (Mourer, 1992). Kraus (1992) suggested using an educational approach that places alcohol treatment within the context of the rehabilitation framework.

Developing Rehabilitation Approaches to Address Areas of Concern for the Disabled Patient

This section addresses a number of areas of life that are vulnerable to stress, particularly when an individual and his or her family are adjusting to the effects of disabilities. Several examples of strategies that can be used to structure rehabilitation practices or communicate informally to people with traumatic injuries and their families are provided.

Self-Worth

Very often, the development of a low sense of self-worth is due to circumstances in childhood and adult life, and the effects of traumatic injury can activate these feelings. A low sense of self-worth is not only a common factor prompting alcohol abuse, but also the most common effect of drinking too much. It is important to understand that the downward spiral that begins when people feel bad about themselves may prompt them to self-medicate to relieve the feelings, and consequently feel worse the following day.

When working with patients, you may suggest that:

- Patients observe and write down the thoughts and feelings they experience prior having the urge to drink. This can assist them in identifying triggers and working on alternative responses to them.
- Patients talk about self-worth issues in support groups or with trusted friends.
- Patients find environments that can provide some of the same positive experiences (companionship, conversation, etc.) that drinking environments once provided.

Coping with Loss

Depression is a common part of the grieving process for people with traumatic injuries and their families. Very often depression and grieving look similar. Some symptoms they have in common include loss of appetite, difficulty sleeping, sadness, worry, negative and critical evaluation of oneself and the world, guilt, blaming, and difficulty or inability to get out of bed or perform everyday functions. Excessive use of alcohol can exacerbate the depression and hinder the grieving process, resulting in losses being unresolved. It is important that patients and their families understand that abusing alcohol will not alleviate the pain, but will simply put it off and give it a chance to grow more intense and cause more problems in everyday life.

Rehabilitation professionals may suggest that, if one feels unable to do anything, forcing oneself to take steps toward some involvement, difficult though it might be at first, will be therapeutic involvement that puts one in the company of people who understand and care, and do not use alcohol or drugs. Caution should be exercised so that the individual does not become excessively involved as energy is usually low during the grieving process, and it can potentially keep one away from the grieving process.

Coping with Anger

Of all of the normal responses to the effects of traumatic injury, anger may be the most difficult to address. Anger is the way humans respond to circumstances and events that they perceive are unfair. Many of the effects of traumatic injury are clearly unfair. These effects often frustrate the basic human desire to believe that life is just. The shift in beliefs that often follows trauma can lead people to become bitter, to deny reality, or to blame themselves or others for things that are not their fault. Alcohol can increase many of the body's anger responses and so increase angry feelings. When alcohol is used to distract oneself from unresolved anger, it is less likely that problems will be solved in an effective way, and more likely that innocent individuals will bear the repercussions.

Suggestions that may assist the patient and family in dealing with anger include:

- Becoming involved in support groups where others have similar experiences and one feels safe discussing anger;
- Pursuing any sort of positive involvement, to affirm that one can have an effect;
- Getting involved in activities that seek to change systems for the better;
- Engaging in activities where one gets a chance to practice arguing, without becoming too emotional on a personal level and losing one's detachment from the subject (i.e., advocacy efforts, debate or discussion groups, etc.);
- Engaging in calming, nondestructive pleasures such as listening to music or playing with pets; or
- Learning relaxation techniques.

Finding Hope and Courage

Feeling vulnerable is frightening. So are pain, change, loss, anger, uncertainty, loss of control, and feelings of entrapment. The combination of these elements can be overwhelming, and can cause an emotional paralysis that compounds the effects of physical or cognitive disabilities. Fear is a natural part of postinjury adjustment for people with traumatic injuries and their families. In understanding fear, it is important to understand that fear often prompts alcohol use. Although at first alcohol might seem to remove fear, in actuality, it increases the level of fear and anxiety.

Suggestions to patients and families may include:

- Talking about one's fears with people who are facing circumstances similar to one's own;
- Seeking out "mentors" who have overcome the types of adversity that are currently sources of fear in one's life;
- Spending as much time as possible around positive people;
- Learning meditation, self-hypnosis, guided imagery, or other practices that will increase the effectiveness of one's affirmation and visualization skills;
- Engaging in activities that involve spiritual people to increase faith and communication on a spiritual level; or
- Engaging in drug-free activities that can serve as temporary distractions from fear, such as movies, music.

Additional Considerations

Drugs

Many drugs are used for relaxation. Like alcohol, most of them are depressants that interfere with mental function and carry a high risk for addiction. The most common are diazepam (Valium), chlordiazepoxide (Librium), alprazolam (Xanax), and lorazepam (Ativan).

When working with alcohol-dependent patients, remember that it may be difficult for the patient to grasp the concept of addiction (Rawson, Obert, & McCann, 1991). The inability to understand addiction can be considered a form of denial; however, from the alcoholic's perspective, the situation is disorienting and confusing.

An important tool in addressing this problem and engaging alcohol-dependent disabled patients in rehabilitation activities is accurate, understandable information. One way for professionals to gain credibility is to be able to give them an explanation for their behavior. The key to this explanation is that the brain has been modified by a substance. It is necessary to convey that alcohol addiction is a true physiological disorder that has changed the way the brain functions (Rawson et al., 1991).

Relaxation training, exercise programs, and practical training in time management improve the quality of life and promote abstinence; many people formerly consumed by the acquisition and use of alcohol are surprisingly unable to structure their free time, and must learn how to enjoy leisure time without alcohol.

The Recovering Patient

Should the refusal of medication by a patient who is in recovery be respected? Absolutely. The decision to take medication should always be the patient's, not the health care team's.

There is considerable discontent with traditional medical facilities among those in recovery because certain medications can threaten sobriety. These drugs include minor tranquilizers, hypnotics, and narcotic analgesics. Persons in recovery often encounter a medical system that continually uses these medications after surgery or illness to supplement other more curative forms of therapy.

Recovering individuals have learned to turn their crisis of active use into a issue of personal growth, accept their health as their responsibility, and see a spiritual component of it. Despite the identification of these special needs, there is very little in thc medical literature to guide the general medical community in treating this growing segment of the population.

If your patient has participated in a treatment program in the past, advise him or her to contact program counselors for advice and support. True, most treatment programs advocate abstinence from all medications that affect consciousness. But their intent is not to make the recovered patient suffer needless discomfort. Most programs suggest alternative methods for handling pain when pain medication may be needed (McCaffery, 1988).

The following are suggestions that you may want to share with the recovering patient that will help during times of illness:

- Contact an AA or NA sponsor or friend;
- If possible, attend meetings more frequently;
- Read 12-step literature, and do not isolate yourself;

- Look for the cause of discomfort and try to treat it—do not just look for symptom relief; and
- Look to nonchemical means of symptom relief, such as relaxation techniques, heat, ice, massage, or rest.

If your patient does not choose to take medication, suggest other forms of pain relief. If necessary, use nonaddictive medications such as aspirin, acetaminophen, ibuprofen, or other nonsteroidal anti-inflammatory agents for pain; antacids, Compazine suppositories for nausea; Kaopectate and Immodium for diarrhea, and so on.

Encourage patients to ask for the cause of the illness and the rationale for the treatment plan, side effects, proper dosage, and the names of any medications prescribed. If a diagnostic procedure or surgery is recommended, encourage them to request an explanation as to what will be done, what preparation is required, and if there are any reasonable alternatives. This provides patients with an opportunity to participate in the decision-making process. Helping patients to maintain a healthy recovery program is the best insurance to prevent relapse in times of illness.

Dietary Guidelines

Diet is perhaps the single most important component to good health. A healthy diet can heal the body and help to correct metabolic problems (Beasley & Knightly, 1994). According to Larson (1994), "just as a healthy nonalcoholic requires proper nourishment for body and mind to function, the victim of alcohol has a vulnerability that requires both a compensating diet and psychological support" (p. 16).

Given the serious damage that alcohol can inflict on nutritional status, and consequently on the rehabilitation process, it is imperative that nutritionists be part of the rehabilitation team. Of paramount importance to the alcohol-dependent disabled patient is the cessation of alcoholic beverages. According to the American Dietetic Association (ADA), nutritional care should include an evaluation of the alcohol's nutritional status at detoxification, supervision of nutritional rehabilitation that encourages normal eating patterns, and provision of nutrition education to assist the patient and significant others develop an eating plan that supports a stable recovery upon discharge to home (ADA, 1990).

Some basic and helpful strategies to help individuals in recovery include the following:

- Emphasize developing sound nutritional habits;
- Limit sweets;
- Recognize food nutrition as a sign of recovery;
- Encourage the patient to eat breakfast every day;
- Offer a variety of foods;
- Suggest that patients take time to enjoy meals;
- Limit coffee to two cups or drink decaffeinated;
- Warn against use of supplements, unless ordered by a physician.

Many debilitating nutritional consequences result from alcohol abuse. During rehabilitation, adequate nutrition makes a difference in the rate and quality of physical recovery, which prepares individuals to function at a higher level.

AFTERCARE

When developing an aftercare plan, it is important to remember that, in addition to the physical challenges these patients will encounter, they will frequently have to deal with other problems after discharge. They may be excluded from, or unable to participate in, training and job opportunities that would allow them to earn sufficient incomes. Also, some may have high medical expenses because of costly treatments, medications, equipment, and prostheses. In addition, these individuals will more often than not deal with prejudices and stigmas. These range from outright discrimination in jobs and facilities to more subtle staring and avoidance by others.

As previously stated, people with disabilities may abuse alcohol and other drugs for all the same reasons as their nondisabled peers. However, the existence of a disability places them at a considerably higher risk.

Risk Factors to Be Considered

Medication Use

People with disabilities often use medication over extended periods of time. The use of two to five concurrent prescribed medications may be average for some disabilities (Moore & Seigel, 1989). Remember that many drugs of abuse also have medical uses, and many individuals are responsible for self-administration, leading to potential misuse among those who use prescribed drugs. Those who use prescribed medication require specialized information on how those drugs influence behavior or interact with alcohol.

Health Concerns or Chronic Pain

The special medical conditions associated with some disabilities can decrease tolerance for alcohol. The problems associated with decreased tolerance include dangerous levels of intoxication, especially when medications are combined with alcohol. There may be a corresponding increase in risk for accidents from alcohol due to preexisting balance, mobility, or vision impairments. Relying on drugs as a primary means of coping with pain increases the likelihood that chemical coping will be perceived as the best way to deal with physical and emotional pain as well (Krupp, 1968).

Peer Group Differences

People with disabilities, especially those who acquired the disability before adulthood, may have less opportunity for association with peer groups. These social limitations can result in gravitation to peer groups that tolerate abuse of alcohol. This also means that people with disabilities may be more vulnerable to alcohol abuse through peer pressure due to lack of social experience or need for acceptance.

Fewer Social Supports

People who experience disabilities tend to have fewer social outlets and have related problems with underutilization of time. Both of these conditions contribute to initiation of alcohol use or to relapse. When a person has fewer social options, it can be difficult to change friends in order to avoid negative influences. There may be greater difficulty in locating sober social settings when attempting recovery from alcohol dependence.

Enabling of Alcohol Use

Family, friends, and professionals may inadvertently encourage people with disabilities to misuse alcohol. Enabling of alcohol abuse is a particular problem for people with disabilities because of societal misunderstandings about issues involved.

Because disabled individuals are at high risk to initiate or resume alcohol misuse, particular attention should be placed on alcohol education. This can include information on medication use, interaction and socialization skills, and learning about independent living options.

Screening and early identification of alcohol misuse or relapse is imperative to better serve those in need, to avoid potential health complications (Moore & Polsgrove, 1989), to reduce the risk of secondary disabilities, and to maintain cost-effective services. The consequences of abuse can be "hidden" behind the disability without most health care professionals even suspecting a problem.

SUMMARY

In summary, alcohol use can affect the rehabilitation management of disabled patients. Knowledge of a patient's alcohol history can be essential in making clinical decisions throughout the course of rehabilitation and aftercare.

Although there is no cure for alcoholism, recovery is possible. Those who choose to remain abstinent and become actively involved in a recovery/rehabilitation program gain self-esteem, self-respect, self-responsibility, and begin the process of accepting their disability. They experience better health and develop alternative means of managing chronic pain, sleep disorders, spasticity, and stress. Many develop more independent lifestyles, become involved in vocational activities, and resolve financial and legal difficulties.

CHAPTER 11

ALCOHOL-MEDICATION INTERACTIONS

- **How Drugs and Alcohol Interact**
- **Specific Interactions**

This topic is presented separately because of its importance in the assessment and management of both hospitalized patients, and those discharged to home. It applies across the continuum of care. It is imperative that health care providers be familiar with alcohol-medication interactions as this information could potentially save the patient's life. As previously reviewed, alcohol impacts the assessment and treatment of trauma patients. The potential interaction of medications with alcohol may lead to an increased risk of illness, injury, or death.

The elderly may be especially likely to mix drugs and alcohol and are at particular risk for the adverse consequences of such combinations. They are also more likely to suffer medication side effects compared with younger persons, and these effects tend to be more severe with advancing age (Gomberg, 1990). (The use of alcohol among the elderly will be discussed in further detail in Chapter 12.)

The Interface Between Alcohol and Aging

How do you know whether alcohol is causing certain medical problems in a patient who drinks, or whether the aging process itself is responsible? More often than not, it is a combination of the two. Aging and alcohol use are both associated with decreased phase I oxidation in the liver, resulting in addictive toxicity. Chronic use increases clinically reported tolerance to alcohol. There is some evidence for increased neural sensitivity to single doses of alcohol with age. It is also true that a given alcohol dose will produce a higher peak blood alcohol level with age. Aging alters the distribution of most substances, including alcohol, and it changes tissue responsiveness in various parts of the body (American Medical Association [AMA], 1995). For example, because elderly persons usually have a lower body water content, a given amount of alcohol can produce more pronounced effects in them than in younger persons (AMA, 1995).

Benzodiazepines that require oxidative metabolism (e.g., diazepam, librium, flurazepan) are of particular concern in the older drinker. Alcohol also enhances acetaminophen toxicity, even in normal doses, an effect potentiated by the "age" related decrease in acetaminophen clearance. Aging also elevates blood levels and enhances central nervous system effects of opiates, while alcohol acutely decreases opiate clearance, compounding opiate toxicity.

HOW DRUGS AND ALCOHOL INTERACT

To exert its desired effect, a drug generally must travel through the bloodstream to its site of action, where it produces some change in an organ or tissue. Alcohol can influence the effectiveness of a drug by altering its availability (Holder, 1992). Typical alcohol-drug interactions include the following (Lieber, 1992): First, an acute dose of alcohol (a single drink or several drinks over several hours) may inhibit a drug's metabolism by competing with the drug for the same set of metabolizing enzymes. This interaction prolongs and enhances the drug's availability and potential for causing harmful side effects. Second, in contrast, chronic (long-term) alcohol ingestion may activate drug-metabolizing enzymes, thus decreasing the drug's availability and diminishing its effects. After these enzymes have been activated, they affect the metabolism of certain drugs for several weeks after cessation of drinking (Guram, Howden, & Holt, 1992). Thus, a recently abstinent chronic drinker may need higher doses of medications than those required by nondrinkers to achieve therapeutic levels of certain drugs. Third, enzymes activated by chronic alcohol consumption transform some drugs into toxic chemicals that can damage the liver or other organs. Fourth, alcohol can magnify the inhibitory effects of sedative and narcotic drugs at their sites of action in the brain. In addition, some drugs affect the metabolism of alcohol, thus altering its potential for intoxication and the adverse effects associated with alcohol consumption (Lieber, 1992) (see Table 11–1).

SPECIFIC INTERACTIONS

Antibiotics. In combination with acute alcohol consumption, some antibiotics may cause nausea, vomiting, headache, and possibly convulsions; among these antibiotics are furazolidone (Furoxone), griseofulvin (Grisactin), metronidazole (Flagyl), and the antimalarial quinacrine (Atabrine) (Lieber, 1992). In addition, acute alcohol consumption decreases the effectiveness of isoniazid, and chronic alcohol use decreases the effectiveness of rifampin (Lieber, 1992).

Anticoagulants. Acute alcohol consumption enhances the effect of warfarin (Coumadin), increasing the patient's risk for life-threatening hemorrhages (Lieber, 1992). Chronic alcohol consumption reduces warfarin's effect, increasing the risk of blood-clotting disorders (Lieber, 1992).

Antidepressants. Alcoholism and depression are frequently associated (Roy, DeJong, Lamparski, George, & Linnoila, 1991), leading to a high potential for alcohol-antidepressants interactions. Alcohol increases the sedative effect of tricyclic antidepressants such as amitriptyline (Elavil) (Dorian et al., 1983; Seppala, Linnoila, & Mattila, 1979); chronic alcohol consumption appears to enhance effects of some tricyclics, while diminishing the effects of others (Rudorfer & Potter, 1987).

A chemical called tyramine, found in some beers and wine, interacts with some antidepressants, such as monoamine oxi-

Table 11–1. Alcohol and Prescription and Nonprescription Medications.

Alcohol Combined With	***Can Cause***
Sleeping medications (e.g., Halcion, Dalmane) Tranquilizers (e.g., Xanax, Valium, Ativan) Antidepressants (e.g., Elavil, Trofanil) Pain relievers (e.g., Percodan, codeine) Some muscle relaxants (e.g., Robaxin, Soma) Antihistamines (e.g., Chlor-Trimeton, Benadryl) Motion-sickness pills (e.g., Dramamine) Allergy medications (e.g., Contac, Dristan) Some cough/cold products Some high blood pressure medications (e.g., Aldomet)	Excessive drowsiness, impaired coordination, mental confusion, rapid intoxication, loss of consciousness, impaired breathing. Can be fatal.
Antianginal medication (e.g., Isordil, nitroglycerin) Some high-blood presssure medications (e.g., Minipress, Apresoline, diuretics)	Dizziness, fainting, lightheadedness, loss of consciousness, falls that could result in physical injury.
Aspirin Antiarthritic medications (e.g., Feldene, Naprosyn, ibuprofen) Potassium tablets Blood thinners (e.g., Coumadin)	Increase in stomach irritation, possible increase in stomach bleeding.
Flagyl Oral antidiabetic medications. Some anti-fungal and antibiotics agents (e.g., Chloromycetin)	Can cause Antabuse-like reaction (weakness, headache, nausea/vomiting, flushing, rapid heartbeat, difficulty breathing)
Antidiabetic medications (e.g., Micronase, insulin) Epilepsy medication (e.g., Dilantin) Gout medication (e.g., Zyloprim)	Interference with control of certain medical conditions (e.g., diabetes, epilepsy, gout). Can cause change in effectiveness of drug treatment.

dase inhibitors, to produce a dangerous rise in blood pressure (Lieber, 1992). This interaction may occur with the consumption of one drink.

Antidiabetic medications. Acute alcohol consumption prolongs and chronic alcohol consumption decreases the effects of tolbutamide (Orinase). It also interacts with some drugs of this class to produce symptoms of nausea and headache (Lieber, 1992).

Antihistamines. Alcohol may intensify the sedation caused by some antihistamines such as Benadryl (Seppala et al., 1979). These drugs may cause excessive dizziness and sedation in older persons; the effects of combining alcohol and antihistamines may therefore be especially significant in this population (Dufour, Archer, & Gordis, 1992).

Antipsychotic medications. Acute alcohol consumption increases the sedative effect of drugs such as chlorpromazine (Thorazine) (Shoaf & Linnoila, 1991) resulting in impaired coordination and potentially fatal breathing difficulties (Lieber, 1992). In addition, the combination of alcohol ingestion and antipsychotic drugs may result in liver damage.

Antiseizure medications. Acute alcohol consumption increases the effects of phenytoin (Dilantin) and the risk of drug-related side effects. Chronic drinking may decrease phenytoin's effects, consequently reducing the patient's protection against epileptic seizures during periods of abstinence (Greenspan & Smith, 1991; Guram et al., 1992).

Antiulcer medications. Some research suggests that a low dose of alcohol increases the effect of cimetidine (Tagamet) and ranitidine (Zantac) in some circumstances; however, this finding remains inconclusive.

Cardiovascular medications. Acute alcohol consumption in combination with some of the medications included in this category can cause dizziness or fainting upon standing up. These include nitroglycerin, reserpine, methyldopa (Aldomet), hydralazine (Apresoline), and guanethidine (Ismeline). In addition, the chronic consumption of alcohol with propranolol (Inderal) reduces its therapeutic effect (Lieber, 1992).

Narcotic pain relievers. As you may recall, this category includes the opiates—morphine, codeine, and meperidine (Demerol), to name a few. The combination of opiates and alcohol enhances the sedative effect of both substances, increasing the risk of death from overdose (Kissin, 1974).

Nonnarcotic pain relievers. Aspirin and similar nonprescription pain relievers are most commonly used by the elderly (Gomberg, 1990). Some of these drugs cause stomach bleeding and inhibit blood from clotting; alcohol can exacerbate these effects (Rees & Turnberg, 1980). Persons who combine alcohol with large doses of aspirin to self-medicate for pain are therefore at particularly high risk for episodes of gastric bleeding. In addition, alcohol may enhance the effects of aspirin (Dufour et al., 1992).

Anesthetics. Chronic alcohol consumption increases the dose of proponfol (Diprivin) required to induce loss of consciousness (Fassoulaki, Farinotti, Servin, & Desmonts, 1993). It also increases the risk of liver damage that may be caused by the anesthetic gases enflurane (Ethrane) (Tsutsumi et al., 1990) and halothane (Fluothane) (Ishii et al., 1983).

Sedatives and hypnotics. Alcohol may cause excessive sedation in the presence of benzodiazepines (Girre, Facy, Lagier, & Dally, 1988). This may be especially true in older people, who demonstrate an increased response to these drugs (Dufour et al., 1992; Gomberg, 1990). Low doses of flurazepam (Dalmane) interact with low doses of alcohol to impair driving ability, even when alcohol is ingested the morning after (Linnoila, Mattila, & Kitchell, 1979). The combination of alcohol and lorazepam (Ativan) may result in depressed heart and respiratory functions; therefore, lorazepam should not be administered to intoxicated patients. In addition, acute alcohol consumption enhances the sedative effects of barbiturates. After detoxification, however, alcoholics may need higher than normal doses of anesthetics and hypnotics, due to cross-tolerance.

It is important to note that, even though barbiturates and tranquilizers may be safe for most nonalcoholics when taken according to a physician's instruction, they can be harmful to an alcoholic. They have the potential of creating a dependence as devastating as dependence on alcohol. Even over-the-counter medications pose a threat to the sobriety of an alcoholic. The alcoholic may have a tendency to misuse, consequently leading to readdiction.

Many reasons contribute to the potential for readdiction. In some cases a drug acts in a similar manner in the body as does alcohol. Such is the case with barbiturates, benzodiazepines, and other medications that act like sedatives. Secondary to the development of a cross-tolerance, the body will respond in the same manner to drugs that are depressants as it will to the consumption of alcohol.

SUMMARY

It is important to remember that a recovering alcoholic's automatic response will be to turn to chemical relief for uncomfortable feelings and to take more than the usual, prescribed amount. It is important to suggest and encourage nonchemical solutions for dealing with the discomforts of everyday living.

CHAPTER 12

ALCOHOL ABUSE AND THE ELDERLY

- **Age of Onset**
- **Barriers to Diagnosis and Treatment**
- **Screening and Assessment**
- **Drug and Alcohol History**
- **Treatment Strategies**

Elderly persons are generally more unstable physically than younger persons, they exhibit lower extremity weakness and decreased balance and vision. Because of their relative physical fragility, they sustain more serious traumatic injuries. The elderly thus constitute a significant proportion of hospitalized trauma patients.

Falls are the leading cause of nonfatal injury, accounting for nearly 800,000 hospitalizations annually; the death rate resulting from falls among people aged 75 and older is nearly 12 times as great as the rate for all ages combined. The elderly are particularly susceptible to falls. Each year an estimated 200,000 older Americans suffer hip fractures associated with falls. Of these, as many as 40,000 die of complications within 6 months and another 40,000 require lifelong nursing home care (Hingson & Howland, 1987). Others are discharged with home care.

Hip and femur fractures are a type of traumatic injury with a higher incidence rate among the elderly. As a result of decreased bone density associated with osteoporosis in postmenopausal women and with aging in general, elderly persons frequently fracture these bones after simple falls.

Although alcoholism has been increasingly diagnosed and treated in the population as a whole, persons aged 60 and over still are a "hidden" group (AMA, 1995). It is estimated that up to 10% of elders living at home and as many as 40% in nursing homes suffer from alcoholism.

In any clinical situation, in hospital settings especially, as many as one of every two elderly patients may be alcoholic. At least 10% of patients in emergency departments who have alcohol-related medical problems are over the age of 60. Even small amounts of alcohol can cause significant motor and cognitive impairments in this group.

Becoming aware that alcoholism exists in the elderly, and that drinking may play a role in trauma incurred by the elderly as well as in the onset and severity of medical disorders, is an important step toward improving health care.

AGE OF ONSET

Alcoholism among the elderly has been differentiated on the basis of age of onset. Early onset alcohol abuse or dependence represents the continuation of lifelong drinking problems, whereas late-onset alcohol abuse or dependence develops after many years during which no problems related to alcohol use were experienced. The latter is less likely to be associated with a family history of alcoholism or psychological disorders and is a milder, more well-defined condition; it also may be more common than originally thought (Atkinson, Tolson, & Turner, 1990). Factors contributing to the development of late-onset drinking problems include increased biological sensitivity to alcohol, late life stresses, more free time, death of friends and loved ones, pressure from peers in some retirement communities to increase alcohol intake, and/or failing health (Alexander & Duff, 1988). The deterioration in this group is very rapid, covering in a year or two the progression seen in alcoholics who have been drinking for 10 to 40 years (Robertson, 1992).

BARRIERS TO DIAGNOSIS AND TREATMENT

Several aspects of aging may interfere with the detection of alcohol use problems among the elderly (Caracci & Miller, 1991; Graham, 1986). For example, younger people may meet DSM-IV criteria for a diagnosis of alcohol abuse or dependence if they persist in drinking, because alcohol use can interfere with their major day-to-day obligations. However, work- and family-related responsibilities are sharply reduced among the elderly, and consequences of alcohol use for these individuals may differ if, for example, they are not well-nourished (Klein & Iber, 1991; Robertson, 1992).

Physiological effects of alcohol may be mistakenly attributed to the aging process, to concomitant chronic disease, or to the side effects of prescription medication (Graham, 1986; Klein & Iber, 1991). Even if alcohol is suspected as the cause of problems or routine alcohol screening is conducted, accurate reporting could be reduced among older individuals who may have memory problems, who may have difficulty answering computational questions related to drinking frequency, or who may be more likely to feel that there is a stigma attached to drinking.

Some families may unthinkingly "encourage" drinking in older family members if they have the attitude that drinking should be tolerated because older people have only a limited time left and, therefore, should be allowed to "enjoy" themselves.

Attitudes toward alcoholism and aging on the part of health care professionals often create obstacles to identification, diagnosis, and treatment of older patients who have drinking problems. Denial is foremost, a hallmark of the disease. It is intensified in many elderly patients who may view alcoholism as a sin or weakness and are reluctant to admit to symptoms. The elderly alcoholic seldom is drunk and disorderly, rarely is arrested for driving while intoxicated, and, though often a victim, is almost never a perpetrator of family violence. Pessimism about treatment outcome, elder discrimination, and the uncertainty about how to address alcohol problems in the elderly may also be barriers.

SCREENING AND ASSESSMENT

As with any other patient being assessed for alcoholism, the following should be considered: the elderly patient's general medical history, including past and present alcohol and other drug use history; living conditions and relationships with family; and friends, and a thorough physical examination. The patient's mental status should also be assessed (AMA, 1995).

In assessing the patient, flexibility is key. Depending on circumstances and the availability of information resources, the assessment process may be changed.

The problems that elderly alcoholics demonstrate include significant impairment in social and interpersonal function, waxing and waning organic mental symptoms, marked behavioral and personality changes, deterioration of interpersonal relationships, proneness to accidents, and deficiencies in self-care capacity (Zimberg, 1985). Other symptoms tend to be nonspecific, including "failure to thrive," insomnia, diarrhea, and dementia. The patient may present with a variety of concerns or complaints such as being worried about drinking, suffering from one or more physiological or psychological complaints or symptoms, being overtly intoxicated or in withdrawal, or coming in for a periodic check-up and possibly being unaware of any major drinking problems (AMA, 1995).

When speaking with patients, you want to put the patient at ease, not on the defensive. It is important to be circumspect in your questioning and discussions. Verbalize that you are interested in the patient's health and ability to function and are not making moral judgments (AMA, 1995).

Morbidity and increased mortality can occur with no more than one or two drinks daily, because of altered pharmacokinetics with aging. Recognizing alcohol-induced brain injury, which can resemble Alzheimer's disease, is particularly important in the management of older patients.

General Medical History

There are clinical clues to help identify active alcoholism in older patients. According to Egbert (1993), signs and/or symptoms that may indicate the presence of alcoholism include:

- Trauma, including frequent falls, accidents, bruises, and fractures;
- Repeated visits to the emergency department;
- Persistent health problems such as hyperuricemia, pancreatitis, gastrointestinal disturbances, and unstable diabetes;

- Insomnia or chronic fatigue related to poor sleeping habits;
- Diarrhea, urinary incontinence, weight loss, or malnutrition;
- Cognitive deterioration, including confusion and memory loss;
- Therapy is not working for a treatable medical illness or disease, such as hypertension;
- Complaints of anxiety (related to undiagnosed withdrawal), with frequent use of or requests for sedatives or hypnotics;
- Presenting signs and/or symptoms of depression; and
- Unexplained postoperative agitation, anxiety, confusion, or new-onset seizures (suggesting withdrawal), especially in patients without known cerebrovascular disease.

Often, elderly patients receiving home care may describe these signs or symptoms to health care professionals, or they may become evident to family members or other professionals. Further evaluation of the patient is warranted when these "clues" appear.

DRUG AND ALCOHOL HISTORY

The elderly consume more medication, both prescription and over-the-counter, than any other age group, and are likely to be forthcoming about such use, even though they may not be able to recall all of the preparations or exact dosages they are taking. There are special risks related to these medications. Older persons living alone may make errors in taking medications (Williams, 1984).

In assessing alcohol consumption, the classic two-question screening test may be used. This includes the following two questions:

- "Have you ever had a drinking problem?"
- "When was your last drink?"

However, it is important to bear in mind that, in response to direct questioning about alcohol, accurate reporting could be reduced among older individuals who have memory problems, may have difficulty answering computational questions related to drinking frequency, or may be more likely than younger persons to feel that there is a stigma attached to drinking. They often look on alcohol as a form of self-medication to help them fall asleep, alleviate pain, or overcome feelings of loneliness or depression.

In the case of the elderly, the absolute quantity of alcohol is not the best indicator; rather, the pattern of use and its physical, psychological, and social effects on the patient's life (AMA, 1995) are more indicative. Accurate information about drinking habits may be very difficult to obtain. Therefore, it may be necessary to question a reliable informant such as a friend or family member in addition to interviewing the patient.

You may also choose to elicit information by utilizing a self-assessment questionnaire. Other options include the Michigan Alcoholism Screening Test—Geriatric Version (MAST-G) (for further information, contact Frederic Blow, Ph.D., at the University of Michigan Alcohol Research Center, 400 E. Eisenhower Pkwy, Suite A, Ann Arbor, MI 48104, 313-998-7952), or the CAGE.

In addition to a drug and alcohol history, details about the patient's living arrangements, family life, employment situation, and recreational activities should also be pursued. Laboratory test results also serve as an indicator of possible alcohol abuse and/or dependency. These may include:

- Blood alcohol level (BAL) of 150 or more without signs of intoxication;
- Possible increase in liver enzyme asparate aminotransferase (LAST);
- Elevation in the serum gamma glutamyltransferase (SGGT); and/or
- Elevation in the mean corpuscular volume (MCV).

Physical Examination

Alcoholism in older patients has a high rate of adverse physical and cognitive consequences. In the Iowa 65+ Rural Heath Survey, elderly heavy drinkers had a significantly higher rate of stroke (17% versus 7% in nondrinkers), peptic ulcer (24% versus 17%), insomnia (21% versus 6%), and urinary incontinence (14% versus 3%) (Colsher & Wallace, 1990).

Health care providers should suspect alcoholism when a physical examination reveals: bruises, abrasions, and scars in locations that might indicate frequent falls; physical altercations or other violent behavior; cigarette burns on the fingers; flushed or florid faces; peripheral neuropathy; hypertension; cirrhosis or other evidence of liver impairment, for example, edema in the lower extremities, and ascites; psoriasis and signs of immunodeficient disorders; as well as other signs previously discussed in Chapter 5.

Age-Related Effects of Alcohol Use

Peripheral neuropathy	Osteopenia
Diminished proprioception	Susceptibility to infection
Alcoholic liver disease	Electrolyte imbalance
Alcoholic pancreatitis	Esophageal varices
Peptic ulcer	Gastritis
Malignancies, especially head, throat, and esophagus	Cardiomyopathy
	Anemia
Malnutrition	Delirium tremens
GI bleeding	Seizures
Hypovitaminosis	Hypertension
Stroke	Organic brain syndrome
Myocardial infarction	Cirrhosis
Respiratory disease	Falls
Fractures	Cognitive deficiencies

Sources: American Medical Association. (1995). *Alcoholism in the Elderly: Diagnosis, Treatment, Prevention—Guideline for Primary Care Physicians.* Chicago, IL: Author; Council on Scientific Affairs. (1996). Alcoholism in the elderly. *Journal of the American Medical Association, 275,* 1–6.

After heavy drinking over a period of many years, liver disease often develops, and most elderly alcoholics with hepatic pathology have cirrhosis. Cancers, especially of the mouth, larynx, and esophagus, are not uncommon in older alcoholic patients, especially those who smoke. Cardiomyopathy and other cardiovascular problems, hypertension and stroke, nutritional deficiencies, impaired sexual function, sleep disorders, and the development of organic brain syndrome also illustrate the combined influence of alcohol and the aging process (AMA, 1995).

Mental Status Examination

The psychological sequelae of the alcohol-aging interface can be as significant as the physiological effects. Clinical studies have shown that a history of drinking is positively associated with dementia as well as other psychiatric disorders, most notably depression (Cook, Winokur, Garvey, & Beach, 1991). It becomes extremely important for the patient's cognitive functioning, emotional affect, and ability to recall recent events to be evaluated to determine whether the depression or other psychiatric disorder is symptomatic of alcoholism, or vice versa, or whether they are in fact coexisting disorders. Alcoholics often display: severe memory loss, an inability to concentrate, defensiveness or irritation when asked general questions about alcohol use, extreme mood swings, undue concern about physical ailments, and suicidal ideation (AMA, 1995).

TREATMENT STRATEGIES

Treatment for alcoholism in the elderly is not that much different from treatment in younger patients, except that special medical and social needs related to aging and frailty often must be taken into account.

The medical consequences of long-term alcohol use can be severe in the older patient and often require immediate attention. Conditions such as internal bleeding, fractures and other trauma resulting from falls, and ischemic events and profound mental confusion are not uncommon, and may be the presenting diagnosis. Other signs and/or symptoms that may require immediate attention include: the effects of central nervous system intoxication, including ataxia and dyskinesia, aspiration pneumonia, loss of consciousness, angina and other cardiac involvement, renal and bladder complications, hypoglycemia, and panic attacks.

Treatment of Alcohol Withdrawal in the Elderly

Withdrawal from alcohol can be a medical emergency, even life-threatening, for older persons, and is generally more severe than in younger patients. Detoxification may take several weeks or even months, and is best initiated in a hospital setting, where the patient and medication can be closely monitored (AMA, 1995). Benzodiazepines, the drugs of choice in acute withdrawal treatment of the elderly, should be administered in doses that are a half to a third of those used for younger patients, because of differences in metabolism and absorption rates. Medications that require hepatic metabolism should be avoided. Ativan and Serax are the drugs of choice for older patients. Clonidine patches (Catapress TTS) are useful in minor to moderate withdrawal and may replace Ativan. Clonidine controls autonomic hyperactivity, anxiety, insomnia, and delirium tremens. Special attention should be paid to monitoring fluids and electrolytes, especially in patients who are taking diuretics. Thiamine therapy should always be instituted to prevent the development of encephalopathy and peripheral neuropathies.

As with younger patients, the severity and duration of withdrawal will vary with the intensity and length of time of the addiction. Persons with late-onset alcoholism tend to have an easier and less complicated withdrawal than patients whose disease is long-standing (AMA, 1995).

During withdrawal, supportive care should be provided. This includes making sure that the patient is well-hydrated, supervising the environment for safety, decreasing stimulation, and providing proper nutrition. Fluids and electrolytes should be monitored and family support is helpful for the patient as it provides a "reality orientation." The patient should rest and can be medicated, but the goal is to sedate the patient while still allowing the patient to be easily aroused.

Following withdrawal treatment, the patient's cognitive status and possible other mental impairments may be more adequately assessed. Those that are not related to the direct effects of alcohol are likely to persist, and need to be addressed during treatment and aftercare.

There are recommended protocols and descriptions of the treatment of alcohol withdrawal; however, each case must be assessed according to its own characteristics with individual signs and symptoms treated accordingly, as required.

Treatment

Once suspected, how do you get an older person to seek treatment? Alcoholics of all ages deny they have a drinking problem. The disease concept of alcoholism was accepted by the AMA in 1956, but these people have never heard of it. When they were growing up, alcoholics were skid-row bums; immoral, weak people (Robertson, 1992). Most were brought up to deal with their emotional problems, and they often view alcoholism as a sin. To overcome this, intervention is necessary.

Intervention involves presenting the facts about alcoholism to the drinker in a tone that is nonjudgmental and shows concern. The goal of intervention is to get the alcoholic to acknowledge the need for help. If detoxification is required, it should be inpatient secondary to the potential medical risks. The suggested approach is to be loving and gentle. The use of words like "drink," "drunkard," or "alcoholic" should be avoided. Those who treat older patients agree that the confrontational approach, which often works well with younger patients, is absolutely wrong for older people (Robertson, 1992). Once in treatment, the late-onset drinker usually responds well. In the Mayo Clinic Study, 25% of older alcoholics were abstinent at one year after treatment (Finlayson, Hurt, Davis, & Morse, 1988).

Effective treatment depends on patient motivation, education, age, gender, family history, social and psychiatric status and chronicity, and duration and severity of the alcohol abuse or dependence. Others factors that can also have an effect are medical problems, legal difficulties, employment situations, and whether the patient abuses other drugs in addition to alcohol.

There are several options, including inpatient facilities, outpatient programs, halfway houses and other residential settings. Much will depend on the patient's health status, financial situation, and social supports (AMA, 1995). Treatment programs that emphasize social relationships and positive aspects of a patient's life have tended to be more successful for elderly drinkers, as opposed to programs that use traditional confrontation and focus on past failures.

The problems of the elderly are often different from those of younger patients and may require specific attention in treatment. They may be experiencing an emotional reaction to retirement, feelings of bereavement from the death of a spouse, and physical pain from illness. Of great importance with the elderly are social issues—isolation, poverty, and boredom. These must be considered in rehabilitation in the older alcoholic. In addition to individual and/or group counseling, family therapy may also be warranted in these cases.

The goal of treatment should be abstinence; however, relapse to drinking and associated harmful behavior is not uncommon in alcoholics and is not necessarily an indication of treatment failure. Ongoing communication and assessment with the patient assists in intervening promptly in the case of relapse and can forestall the development of another acute stage of the disease as well as new medical complications (AMA, 1995).

In encouraging the patient to become and remain abstinent, Alcoholics Anonymous (AA) and similar support groups can be of assistance during the immediate postdetoxification period, as well as in long-term treatment (Hinmichsen, 1990). In AA, one third of the members are over the age of 50; older alcoholics respond better to age-specific groups and socialization.

Referral

As with other patients, involvement in an aftercare program is indicated in most cases. Although some older people are able to go into remission from alcoholism without formal treatment, most, if left to their own devices, will return to former drinking habits after a brief period of abstinence.

Many communities have a range of alcoholism treatment facilities and programs available. You should become acquainted with what is available and select the program equipped to offer the services your elderly patient needs to address his or her specific problems and circumstances.

SUMMARY

There are several key concepts to keep in mind regarding alcoholism in older patients. Alcoholism remains a significant problem in the older population, despite the decline in alcohol use with age. Denial is a major problem in alcoholism for the patient, family, and health care professionals. Much of the time the disease is misdiagnosed, undertreated, and more frequently missed or ignored, especially in older adults who complain of vague symptoms such as depression, urinary problems, diarrhea, poor appetite, decreased ADL (activity of daily living), self-neglect, falls, and dementia. Because of denial, the patient hides the symptoms of a potentially fatal disease.

The lifestyle of many older adults adds to the difficulty of early identification and intervention. Many of them live alone, they are retired, so job performance is not a problem, and they often do not drive. Hidden drinking often continues without interruption.

Alcoholism has more adverse physical and cognitive consequences in older patients than younger patients. Alcoholism may not even begin until old age. Left untreated, the prognosis for alcoholism in the elderly patient is poor and more likely to be fatal.

APPENDIX A

ALCOHOL AND OTHER DRUGS ASSESSMENT AND SCREENING INSTRUMENTS

The following is a partial listing of Alcohol and Other Drugs Assessment and Screening Instruments.

Addiction Severity Index (ASI)
National Clearinghouse for Alcohol and Drug Abuse Information
PO Box 2345
Rockville, MD 20847-2345
800-729-6686
301-468-2600

The ASI is a structured, 45-minute clinical research interview to assess problem severity in seven areas commonly affected by addiction: medical condition, illegal activity, alcohol and other drug abuse, employment and income, family and social relations, and psychiatric status (Soucy, Kelly, & Cardenas, 1994).

Adolescent Drinking Index
Psychological Assessment Resources, Inc.
PO Box 998
Odessa, FL 33556
1-800-331-TEST

This is a 24-item self-reporting rating scale intended to measure the severity of drinking problems (Hoshino, 1992; McLellan & Dembo, 1992).

Adolescent Drinking Inventory Psychological Assessment Resources, Inc. PO Box 998 Odessa, FL 33556 1-800-331-TEST	This is a 25-question self-report instrument that focuses on drinking-related loss of control and social, psychological, and physical symptoms of alcohol problems.
Alcohol Dependence Scale (ADS) Addiction Research Foundation 33 Russell St. Toronto, Ontario M5S-2S1, Canada 1-800-661-1111	This is a 25-item questionnaire. It is derived from the Alcohol Use Inventory. It yields an index of severity of alcohol dependence (Crist & Milby, 1990; NIAAA, 1990; Horn, Skinner, Wanberg, & Foster, 1984).
Alcohol Expectancy Questionnaire Dr. Mark Goldman Alcohol and Drug Abuse Research Institute Department of Psychology, BEH 339 University of South Florida Tampa, FL 33620 813-974-6963	Used to gauge high risk circumstances that may lead to alcohol use (NIAAA, 1991).
Alcohol Use Disorder Identification Test (AUDIT)	This 10-item questionnaire provides information on alcohol use, dependence, and problems resulting from drinking during the past year. The AUDIT takes approximately 2 minutes to administer (Babor & Grant, 1989).
American Drug and Alcohol Survey (ADAS) RMBSI, Inc. 2100 W. Drake Rd. Suite 144 Fort Collins, CO 80526 1-800-447-6354	This 57-item survey requires 20 to 25 minutes to complete. It develops a typology of nine styles of use of drugs that are listed in order of increasing severity of drug involvement (McLellan & Dembo, 1992).
Beck Depression Inventory The Psychological Corporation Order Service Center PO Box 839954 San Antonio, TX 78283-3954 800-228-0752	The BDI is a well-established, brief questionnaire is easily used to assess symptoms of depression. The BDI is self-administerd and easily scored, and the results are widely recognized.

CAGE Questionnaire

A self-report screening consisting of four yes-no questions. Requires approximately 1 minute to complete (Ewing, 1984; NIAAA, 1990).

Chemical Dependency Assessment Profile (CDAP)
Multi-Health Systems (MHS) and Publishers
908 Niagara Falls Blvd.
North Tonawanda, NY 14120
1-800-456-3003

This 235-item multiple-choice self-report instrument assesses alcohol and other drug use and chemical dependency problems (McLellan & Dembo, 1992).

Chemical Use, Abuse and Dependence Scale (CUAD)

The CUAD is a brief semistructured interview designed to assess problems with all drugs of abuse. It determines a severity score of each drug used, and total severity score that considers the overall profile. It is at minimum a 2-item and at maximum an 80-item scale (McGovern & Morrison, 1992).

Clinical Institute Withdrawal Assessment (CIWA)

This tool aids in quantifying the signs and symptoms of withdrawal in the alcohol abuser; the values obtained are used to guide medical personnel in medication administration to ensure a safe and comfortable detoxification for patients.

Comprehensive Addiction Severity Index for Adolescents (CASI-A)
Kathleen Meyers
Penn/V.A. Center for Studies of Addiction
PVAMC Building 7
University & Woodland Aves.
Philadelphia, PA 19104
215-823-5809

This structured interview was designed to evaluate drug and alcohol use and psychosocial severity in adolescent populations in a variety of settings. It is administered by an assessor; it takes approximately 50 to 60 minutes to complete.

Comprehensive Drinker Profile (CDP)
Psychological Assessment Resources
PO Box 998
Odessa, FL 33556
1-800-331-TEST

This is a 99-item structured interview questionnaire. It is designed to provide a history of drinking practice and problems. It incorporates the MAST and requires from 1 to 2 hours to administer (Crist & Milby, 1990).

Health Screening Survey (HSS)	This is a 10-item masked screening instrument consisting of the CAGE questions, questions about frequency and quantity of use, history of use and problems, and the Skinner Trauma Scale (Wallace & Haines, 1985).
Inventory of Drinking Situations Addiction Research Foundation 33 Russell Street Toronto, Ontario, M5S-2S1, Canada 1-800-661-1111	Used to identify emotional, cognitive, and social factors that may precipitate drinking (NIAAA, 1991).
Michigan Alcoholism Screening Test (MAST) Melvin L. Selzer 4016 Third Ave. San Diego, CA 92103 619-299-4043	Quantifies the severity of alcohol problems for adults, using a 24-item self-administered questionnaire calling for yes or no responses (Crist & Milby, 1990; Tarter, Ott, & Mezzich, 1991).
Personal Experience Screening Questionnaire (PESQ) Western Psychological Services 12031 Wilshire Blvd. Los Angeles, CA 90025 310-478-1061	This is a 40-item self-report screening questionnaire for use with adolescents suspected of abusing alcohol or other drugs. It takes approximately 10 minutes to administer.
Quantitative Inventory of Alcohol Disorders (QIAD)	This 22-item self-report instrument assesses the severity of alcohol problems during the month before administration of the test. It takes 10–12 minutes to complete (McLellan & Dembo, 1992; Ridley & Kordinak, 1988).
RAFFT	A self-report questionnaire consisting of five questions which could be used in "screening" adolescent patients for risk of substance abuse (Riggs & Alario, 1989).
Self-Administered Alcoholism Screening Test (SAAST)	This is a 34-item questionnaire with a yes-no format; there is also an abbreviated 9-item version. Considered useful for screening medical patients for alcoholism (NIAAA, 1990; Swenson & Morse, 1975).

Short Michigan Alcohol Screening Test (SMAST)	This is a 13-item questionnaire to identify alcohol problems. It reviews an individual's drinking habits, history, and alcohol-related problems. It takes approximately 15 minutes to complete (Selzer, Vinokur, & van Rooijen, 1975; Singer, 1992).
Simple Screening Instrument for AOD Abuse (SSI) National Clearinghouse for Alcohol and Drug Abuse Information PO Box 2345 Rockville, MD 20847-2345 800-729-6686 301-468-2600	This is a 16-item questionnaire that provides a comprehensive screen for alcohol and other drug abuse. The SSI also has a clinical observation checklist for signs and symptoms of AOD abuse.
Skinner Trauma History	This consists of five questions regarding the individual's previous trauma history. A score of two or more positive responses to the five questions has been shown to indicate a high probability of excessive drinking or alcohol abuse (Skinner et al., 1984).
Structured Clinical Interview (SCID) American Psychiatric Press, Inc. 1400 K Street, NW, 11th Floor Washington, DC 20005 1-800-368-5777	This clinical interview is used to assess psychiatric and substance abuse-related disorders. It guides an experienced mental health clinician through all of the major mood, anxiety, psychotic, and substance use disorders (Kleber, 1994).
T-ACE Questionnaire	This instrument is designed to identify pregnant women who consume quantities of alcohol that potentially can damage the fetus. It takes approximately 1 minute to complete and incorporates three items from the CAGE Questionnaire. In addition, it assesses alcohol tolerance (NIAAA, 1990; Sokol, Martier, & Anger, 1989).

APPENDIX B

RESOURCE LIST

ADDITIONAL SOURCES FOR INFORMATION

The organizations included in the following list do not represent an exhaustive exploration of available resources, nor does incorporation in this list represent an endorsement of a particular organization.

Abbott Northwestern Hospital/Sister Kenny Institute
Chemical Dependency/Physical Disability Program
1800 First Avenue, South
Minneapolis, MN 55403
(612) 863-1500

Addiction Intervention with the Disabled (AID)
Sociology Department
Kent State University
Kent, OH 44242
(216) 672-2440

Adult Children of Alcoholics (ACA) World Services
PO Box 3216
252 Sepulveda Boulevard
Torrance, CA 90505
(310) 534-1815

Al-Anon Inter-Group
200 Park Avenue South, Room 814
New York, NY 10159-0182
(212) 254-7236

Alcohol and Drug Problem Association of North America
444 N. Capitol Street, NW, Suite 706
Washington, DC 20001
(202) 737-4340

Alcohol Research Information Service
1106 E. Oakland
Lansing, ME 48906
(517) 485-9900

Alcoholics Anonymous (AA) World Services, Inc.
475 Riverside Drive
New York, NY 10115
(212) 554-0656

American Council on Alcoholism
5024 Campbell Boulevard., Suite H
Baltimore, MD 21236
(301) 529-9200

American Council for Drug Education
6193 Executive Boulevard
Rockville, MD 20850
(301) 984-5700

American Medical Association
515 North State Street
Chicago, IL 60610
(312) 464-5000

American Society of Addiction Medicine
4601 North Park Avenue
Chevy Chase, MD 20815
(301) 656-3920

Association on Higher Education and Disability
P.O. Box 21192
Columbus, OH 43221-0192
(614) 488-4972

BACCHUS of the U.S.
(Boost Alcohol Consciousness Concerning the
Health of University Students)
P.O. Box 10430
Denver, CO 80210
(303) 871-3068

Center for Alcohol and Addiction Studies
Brown University
Box G-BH
Providence, RI 02912
(401) 444-1800

Center for Alcohol Studies
Rutgers University
PO Box 969
Piscataway, NY 08854-0969
(908) 445-2190

Center for Substance Abuse Prevention and Center for Substance Abuse Treatment
Division of State Programs
Rockwall II Building, 6th Floor
5600 Fishers Lane
Rockville, MD 20857
(301) 443-3820

Center for Substance Abuse Prevention National Resource Center for the Prevention of Perinatal Abuse of Alcohol and Other Drugs
9300 Lee Highway
Fairfax, VA 22031
1-800-354-8824

Centers for Disease Control and Prevention
1600 Clifton Road
Atlanta, GA 30333
(404) 639-3824

Children of Alcoholics Foundation, Inc.
Box 4185, Grand Central Station
New York, NY 10115
(800) 359-COAF or (212) 754-0656

Congress on Chemical Dependency and Disability, Inc.
15519 Crenshaw Boulevard, Suite 209
Gardena, CA 90249
(213) 679-6523

Families Anonymous, Inc.
P.O. Box 528
Van Nuys, CA 90274
(818) 989-7841

Hazelden Educational Services
P.O. Box 176
15251 Pleasant Valley Road
Center City, MN 55012-0176
1-800-328-9000

Institute of Black Chemical Abuse
2616 Nicollet Avenue
Minneapolis, MN 55408
(612) 871-7878

Johnson Institute
7151 Metro Boulevard, Suite 250
Minneapolis, MN 55439-2122
1-800-247-0484

Join Together
441 Stuart Street, 6th Floor
Boston, MA 02116
(617) 437-1500

Just Say No Foundation
1777 North California Boulevard, Room 210
Walnut Creek, CA 94596
(415) 939-6666 or 1-800-258-2766

March of Dimes Birth Defects Foundation
PO Box 1657
Wilkes-Barre, PA 18703-1657
1-800-367-6630

Mothers Against Drunk Driving (MADD)
669 Airport Freeway, Suite 310
Hurst, TX 76053
(817) 268-6233

National Acupuncture Detoxification Association
349 East 140th Street
Bronx, NY 10454
(718) 993-3100
or
3115 Broadway #51
New York, NY 10027
(201) 783-3772

National AIDS Information Clearinghouse
PO Box 6603
Rockville, MD 20849-6003
(English) 1-800-458-5231 or (Spanish) 1-800-344-SIDA

National Asian/Pacific American Families Against Substance Abuse, Inc. (NAPAFASA)
6303 Friendship Court
Bethesda, MD 20817
(301) 530-0945

National Association for Children of Alcoholics
11426 Rockville Pike, Suite 100
Rockville, MD 20852
(301) 468-0985
or
31582 Coast Highway, Suite B
South Laguna, CA 92677
(714) 499-3889

National Association for Perinatal Addiction Research and Education
100 North Michigan Avenue, Suite 300
Chicago, IL 60601
(312) 541-1272

National Black Alcoholism and Addictions Council
1629 K Street, NW, Suite 802
Washington, DC 20006
(202) 296-2696

National Clearinghouse for Alcohol and Drug Information
PO Box 2345
Rockville, MD 20847-2345
(301) 468-2600 or 1-800-729-6686

National Coalition of Hispanic Health and Human Services Organizations
1030 15th Street, NW, Suite 1053
Washington, DC 20005
(202) 371-2100

National Coalition on Alcohol and Drug Dependent Women and Their Children
1511 K Street, NW, Suite 926
Washington, DC 10005

National Council on Alcoholism and Drug Dependence (NCADD)
12 West 21st Street, 7th Floor
New York, NY 10010
(212) 206-6770 or 1-800-622-2255

National Drug Information Center of Families in Action, Inc.
2296 Henderson Mill Road, Suite 204
Atlanta, GA 30345
(404) 934-6364

National Head Injury Foundation (NHIF)
1776 Massachusetts Avenue, NW, Suite 100
Washington, DC 20036
(202) 296-6443 or 1-800-444-NHIF

National Institute on Alcohol Abuse and Alcoholism
600 Executive Boulevard, Suite 505
Rockville, MD 20892-7003
(301) 443-1206

National Institute on Disability and Rehabilitation
Research/Model Spinal Cord Injury Systems
Switzer Memorial Building - Room 3430
Washington, DC 20202-2701
(202) 205-9194

National Institute on Drug Abuse
Division of Clinical & Service Research
Medical Affairs Branch
Parklawn Building, Room 10A 12
5600 Fishers Lane
Rockville, MD 20857
(301) 443-4877

National Institute on Neurological Disorders and Stroke
Building 31, Room 8A06
9000 Rockville Pike
Bethesda, MD 20892
(301) 496-5924

National Library of Medicine
Reference Service Division
Videocassette Loan Program
8600 Rockville Pike
Bethesda, MD 20209
(301) 496-4244

National Maternal and Child Health Clearinghouse
8201 Greensboro Drive, Suite 600
McLean, VA 22101
(703) 821-8955, ext. 254

National Organization on Fetal Alcohol Syndrome
1815 H Street, NW, Suite 750
Washington, DC 20006
(202) 785-4585

National Prevention Network
444 North Capitol Street, NW, Suite 642
Washington, DC 20001
(202) 783-6868

National Rehabilitation Information Center
8455 Colesville Road, Suite 935
Silver Springs, MD 22091
1-800-34-NARIC

National Self Help Clearinghouse
33 West 42nd Street
New York, NY 10036

National Spinal Cord Injury Association
600 West Cummings Park, Suite 2000
Woodburn, MA 01801
1-800-962-9629

National Stroke Association
300 East Hampden Avenue, Suite 240
Englewood, CO 80110
(303) 762-9922

National Women's Christian Temperance Union
1730 Chicago Avenue
Evanston, IL 60201
(312) 864-1396

Office of Minority Health Resource Center
PO Box 37337
Washington, DC 20013-7337
1-800-444-6472

Pacific Institute of Chemical Dependency
1188 Bishop Street, Suite 1701
Honolulu, HI 96813
(808) 526-2841

Parents Resource Institute for Drug Education
The Hurt Building
50 Hurt Plaza, Suite 210
Atlanta, GA 30303
(404) 577-4500

Rehabilitation Institute of Chicago
Office of Education and Training
448 E. Ontario, Suite 650
Chicago, IL 60611

Rehabilitation Research and Training Center on Severe Traumatic Brain Injury
Box 434 MCV Station
Richmond, VA 23298-0434
(804) 828-1851

Rehabilitation Research and Training Center on Substance Abuse and Disability
Department of Community Health
School of Medicine
Wright State University
Dayton, OH 45435
(513) 259-1384

Resource Center on Substance Abuse Prevention and Disability
1331 F Street, NW, Suite 800
Washington, DC 20004
(202) 783-2900

Spinal Cord Society
Wendall Road
Fergus Falls, MD 56537
(218) 739-5252

Spinal Network
PO Box 4126
Boulder, CO 80306
(303) 449-5412 or 1-800-338-5412

Substance Abuse and Mental Health Administration
5600 Fishers Lane
Rockville, MD 20857
(301) 443-6315

Substance Abuse Librarians and Information Specialists (SALIS)
Alcoholism and Drug Abuse Institute Library
3937 15th Avenue, ND, NL-15
Seattle, WA 98195
(206) 543-0937

The Institute for Rehabilitation and Research Database of Educational Research on Spinal Cord Injuries
Division of Education
1333 Moursund
Houston, TX 77030
(713) 797-5945

The NADA Literature Clearinghouse
PO Box 1927
Vancouver, WA 98668-1927
(206) 254-0186

ALCOHOL AND OTHER DRUG DATABASES

CORK
Project Cork Resource Center
Dartmouth Medical School
Hanover, NH 03756-3851
(603) 650-1122

QUICK FACTS
CSR, Inc.
1400 Eye Street, NW, Suite 200
Washington, DC 20005
(202) 842-7600

Welch Medical Library
Johns Hopkins University
1900 E. Monument Street
Baltimore, MD 20225
(410) 955-3410

GLOSSARY

Abstinence—The total avoidance of any substance of abuse; the state of being free of alcohol and of all other drugs of abuse.

Acetaldehyde—The initial breakdown product of alcohol in the body.

Acetylcholine—A neurotransmitter found in the cerebral cortex and parasympathetic nervous system.

Acne rosacea—Redness and swelling of the nose and cheeks which is often seen in long-term alcohol dependent persons.

Acquired Immunodeficiency Syndrome (AIDS)—The breakdown of the body's immune system, resulting in the ability to resist infection. There is no cure, and it is almost invariably fatal. AIDS is highly contagious through transmission of the HIV virus which is present in all bodily fluids.

Acute abstinence syndrome—The aggregate of withdrawal signs and symptoms that occur shortly after a person who is physically dependent on a drug stops taking it. The adjective "acute" distinguishes this variant from the "protracted" or "chronic" drug withdrawal or abstinence syndrome.

Acute psychosis—A disturbance in thinking that is often accompanied by delusions and visual or auditory hallucinations. An acute psychosis may be caused by alcohol or other drug withdrawal, drug toxicity (most commonly in conjunction with abuse of cocaine, methamphetamine, or psychedelic agents), or schizophrenia.

Addiction—Physiological and/or psychological dependence on a drug. The overpowering physical or emotional urge to do something repeatedly that an individual cannot control, accompanied by a tolerance for the drug and withdrawal symptoms if the drug use is discontinued. (*See also* Psychological dependence). Alcohol and/or drugs become the central focus of life.

Adrenaline—A trademark for epinephrine, an adrenergic agent.

Aftercare—In alcohol and other drug addiction rehabilitation, the package of services offered clients after completion of a short-term intensive (after residential) treatment program.

Agitation—A restless inability to keep still. Agitation is most often psychomotor agitation, that is, having emotional and physical components. Agitation can be caused by anxiety, overstimulation, or withdrawal from depressants and stimulants.

Alcohol (ethyl)—The intoxicating chemical found in liquors, which is produced by the action of yeast on sugars and starches. Often referred to as "beverage alcohol" as opposed to methyl alcohol which is not consumable and is primarily used for industrial purposes. Alcohol is classified as a central nervous (CNS) system depressant.

Alcohol abuse—Pattern of excessive and/or inappropriate alcohol use distinguishable from addiction by the degree of free choice the individual has in when (or whether) to start or stop use.

Alcohol-induced heart muscle disease—A disease of the heart muscle characterized by irregular rhythms; it is caused by alcohol abuse.

Alcoholic—Individual who has experienced physical, psychological, social, and spiritual deterioration as a consequence of regular and/or excessive use of alcohol. The term *alcoholic* has been variously defined at different times and by different people. However three aspects of the alcoholic have generally been agreed on:

- Their drinking pattern is incompatible with what is expected by the other members of society.
- They have an urge to drink or to continue drinking once they start that they cannot control.
- Their drinking creates either social, economic, or health problems for themselves, their family, and/or society.

Alcoholic dementia—An organic brain syndrome associated with prolonged, heavy ingestion of alcohol, characterized by impairment of long- and short-term memory, abstract thinking and judgment, and other disturbances of higher brain function.

Alcoholism—As defined in the Uniform Act, alcoholism means an illness characterized by habitual lack of self-control as to the consumption of alcoholic beverages or the consumption of alcoholic beverages to the extent that a person's health is substantially impaired or endangered or his or her social and economic function is substantially disrupted.

Alzheimer's disease—A presenile dementia sometimes beginning at middle age and affecting the nerve cells containing acetylcholine located in the frontal and temporal lobes of the cerebrum. Among its effects are speech defects and progressive loss of mental faculties.

Amenorrhea—Abnormal absence or suppression of menstruation.

Amnesia—Memory loss.

Amphetamine—A drug that stimulates the central nervous system, alleviates fatigue, and produces a feeling of alertness and well-being.

Amygdala—A small segment of a lobe found in the cerebellum.

Analgesia—Relief from pain; the state of insensibility to pain without loss of consciousness.

Anemia—Abnormally low number of red blood cells or hemoglobin.

Anesthetic—A substance that causes loss of consciousness and insensibility to pain.

Anorexia—Diminished appetite; aversion to food.

Antabuse (disulfiram)—A drug that interferes with the normal metabolism of alcohol so that a person who drinks after taking disulfiram becomes very ill.

Anterograde amnesia—Inability to learn and form new memories.

Antidepressants—A group of drugs used in treating depressive disorders.

Antipsychotics—A group of drugs used to treat psychotic disorders; sometimes referred to as major tranquilizers or neuroleptics.

Antisocial personality disorder—A pervasive pattern of disregard for, and violation of, the rights of others. The disorder is characterized in part by risk-taking, criminality, and pathological lying.

Anxiety disorders—A group of disorders characterized by unrealistic fear, panic, or avoidance behavior. These disorders include (among others) panic attacks, phobias, obsessive-compulsive disorder, and generalized anxiety disorder.

Arrhythmias—Heart rhythm disturbances.

Ascites—Abnormal accumulation of fluid in the abdominal cavity, sometimes resulting in abdominal distension.

Assessment—The process of collecting detailed information about a person's alcohol and other drug use, emotional and physical health, family and social problems, roles and supports, educational and employment status, legal status, and other areas as a basis for identifying the appropriate level and intensity of alcohol and other drug treatment as well as needs for other services.

Assessment tool—*See* Instrument.

Ataxia—Unsteady walking or staggering, caused by an inability to coordinate the muscles.

Arteriosclerosis—A chronic disease characterized by abnormal thickening and hardening of the arterial walls with resulting loss of elasticity.

Atherosclerosis—Deposition of materials, often fat droplets, in the walls of the arteries, usually leading to narrowing and hardening of the artery wall.

Atherosclerotic narrowing—Thickening and hardening of the medium- and large-sized coronary arteries, usually due to the formation of plaques (fat deposits).

Atrophy—Wasting away, or shrinkage, of tissue, caused by cell death rather than shrinkage of individual cells.

Autonomic nervous system—System of nerves controlling many internal processes, such as heart rate, gastrointestinal activity, pupil diameter, etc.

Axon—Part of a neuron consisting of a single fiber that carries nerve impulses from the neuron to other cells.

Axon terminal—A bulge at the distal end of the axon that contains the synaptic vesicles which enclose the neurotransmitter.

Basal Ganglia—A group of nerve cell structures at the base of the cerebral hemispheres that are involved in motor control.

Barbiturate—A chemical derivative of barbituric acid which will produce a calming effect, as well as sleep, and which is capable of producing mental and/or physical dependence with prolonged or frequent use.

Benzodiazepine—The chemical class of sedative-hypnotic drugs that are used as sedatives and some types are used as sleeping pills. This class includes diazepam (Valium), lorazepam (Ativan), chlordiazepoxide (Librium), etc.

Binge drinking—The consumption of five or more drinks in a row on at least one occasion.

Biopsychosocial—A holistic approach to assessment and treatment that takes into account a person's medical (biological), psychological, and social needs. This approach reflects the understanding that addiction affects the whole person and is influenced by a wide range of factors.

Blackout—A type of memory impairment that occurs when a person is conscious but cannot remember the blackout period. In general, blackouts consist of periods of amnesia or memory loss, typically caused by chronic, high-dose AOD abuse. Blackouts are most often caused by sedative-hypnotics such as alcohol and the benzodiazepines.

Blood brain barrier—A membrane that separates brain tissue from circulating blood; the membrane that impedes transfer of many substances from the bloodstream into brain tissue.

Borderline personality disorder—A disorder beginning in early adulthood that features a pattern of unstable self-image, moods, and interpersonal relationships and occurs in a variety of contexts.

Bradycardia—Relatively slow heart rate.

Brainstem—A stalklike part of the brain that links the base of the brain to the spinal cord.

Brewing—The fermentation of grains that results in beer or ale.

CAGE Questionnaire—A brief alcoholism screening tool asking subjects about attempts to Cut down on drinking, Annoyance over other's criticism of the subject's drinking, Guilt related to drinking, and use of an alcoholic drink as an Eye opener.

Carcinogen—A cancer-causing chemical or agent.

Cardiac disease—Disease affecting the heart.

Cardiomyopathy—A group of diseases of the heart characterized by the inability of the heart muscle cells to contract normally.

Cardiovascular disease—Disease of the heart or blood vessels comprising several disorders, including coronary artery disease, cardiomyopathy, hypertension, hemorrhagic stroke syndrome, and heart rhythm disturbances.

Carotid bruits—An abnormal sound or murmur heard over the carotid artery when listening for sounds produced within the body.

Cerebellum—The brain structure at the base of the brain that is involved in the control of muscle tone, balance, and sensorimotor coordination.

Cerebral Blood Flow (CBF)—Refers to the flow of blood through the brain.

Cerebral cortex—The outer layer of gray matter covering the cerebrum. It contains areas for processing sensory information and for controlling motor functions, speech, higher cognitive functions, emotions, behavior, and memory.

Cerebral hemorrhage—Rupture of a blood vessel in the cerebrum.

Cerebrovascular accident—An occurrence of sudden damage to the brain or to the brain tissue and the blood vessels surrounding it.

Cerebrum—The largest portion of the brain; includes the cerebral hemispheres (cerebral cortex and basal ganglia).

Chemical dependence—Involves loss of control, compulsion to use, continued use against one's own best interests, and in spite of risk and adverse consequences, a belief in the efficacy of drugs, denial of a problem and the need to abstain from all mood-changing, addicting drugs for permanent recovery.

Cholesterol—The most abundant of the naturally occurring steroid molecules (a subclass of lipid, or fat molecules having a common structure); a constituent of many body components, such as hormones and vitamin D, and often associated with the lipoproteins in compounds such as high-density lipoproteins (HDL) and low-density lipoproteins (LDL).

Cirrhosis—The replacement of liver tissue with scar tissue due either to malnutrition and/or excessive and prolonged alcohol use; a chronic liver disease marked by scarring of liver tissue and eventually liver failure.

Cocaine—The primary psychoactive ingredient in the cocoa plant; functions as a behavioral stimulant. Can be snorted, smoked, or injected.

Cognition—Cognitive mental processes. Conscious intellectual activity such as thinking, reasoning, remembering, imagining, or learning.

Cognitive reframing—A relapse prevention skill training strategy that helps the drug-dependent patient find new responses to high-risk factors.

Confabulation—The inventing of tales and readiness to produce answers without regard to facts.

Confidentiality—Anonymity of participants in alcohol- and drug-abuse treatment programs is strictly protected by federal and various individual state regulations.

Congestive heart failure—Progressive inability of a diseased heart to pump sufficient blood to meet the demands of the body.

Coping imagery—A therapeutic technique in which the therapist leads the patient through an alternating series of images, one set pleasant and the other anxiety-provoking, to reduce anxiety by associating the anxiety-provoking situation with a pleasant image.

Coronary artery disease—Disease (such as myocardial infarction or heart attack) resulting from restriction or interruption of the blood supply to the heart muscle via the coronary arteries.

Corpus callosum—The tract of myelin-coated nerve fibers connecting the two cerebral hemispheres.

Corpus striatum—One of the basal ganglia; located deep in the cerebral hemispheres and upper brain stem and involved in the programming of movement; a part of the extrapyramidal system containing the caudate nucleus.

Continuing care—Twelve-step self-help groups, counseling, follow-up, and individualized support for clients following treatment for abuse and addiction.

Convulsions—A seizure is a sudden episode of uncontrolled electrical activity in the brain. If the abnormal electrical activity spreads throughout the brain, the result may be a loss of consciousness and a grand mal seizure. One symptom of a seizure is *convulsions* or twitching and jerking of the limbs. Seizures may occur as the result of head injury, infection, cerebrovascular accidents, withdrawal from sedative-hypnotic drugs, or high doses of stimulants.

Cortex—The outer, convoluted layer of brain tissue; the gray matter.

Crack—Cocaine (cocaine hydrochloride) that has been chemically modified so that it will become a gas vapor when heated at relatively low temperatures; also called "rock" cocaine. "Crack" refers to the crackling sound made when the mixture is heated.

Craving—A term implying both physiological and psychological dependence; the user's "desire" or "need" to continue using a drug. This term is often associated with withdrawal and is considered by some to be a defining characteristic of addiction.

Cue exposure—A cognitive-behavioral intervention that employs gradual exposure to cues to desensitize the drug-dependent patient to those cues.

Cushing's syndrome—A group of symptoms caused by overactivity of the adrenal glands.

Delirium—A state of mental confusion characterized by difficulty in responding to stimuli and an absence of orientation to place and time. May be accompanied by auditory, visual, or tactile hallucinations. May be caused by drug withdrawal or severe intoxication with phencyclidine.

Delirium tremens—A serious and sometimes fatal condition; a state of confusion accompanied by trembling and vivid hallucinations. Symptoms may include restlessness, agitation, uncontrollable shaking (tremors), terror, sleeplessness, rapid heartbeat, fever, and possible convulsions. Delirium tremens often occurs in chronic alcoholics after withdrawal or abstinence from alcohol. Commonly called "DTs."

Delusions—Fixed, irrational ideas not shared by others and not responding to a logical argument.

Dementia—A global intellectual impairment due to organic or emotional causes that includes loss of abstract thinking and memory functions, personality changes, breakdown of social skills, and other disturbances of higher brain functions.

Dendrite—Single or multiple fibers extending from the cell body that branch into treelike structures. They receive chemical information from the axons of other neurons.

Denial—Inability to acknowledge the reality of growing alcohol/drug dependency or its consequences. A psychological defense mechanism.

Depressant—Any chemical that diminishes the activity of the central nervous system, usually resulting in dulled reflexes, impaired thought processes, sleep, and distorted perceptions when taken in large amounts.

Depression—Depressed mood or the loss of interest or pleasure in activities. Symptoms include decreased energy, feelings of worthlessness, appetite disturbance, weight change, feelings of inappropriate or excessive guilt, psychomotor agitation or retardation, difficulty thinking or concentrating, recurring thoughts of death or suicide, or suicide attempts.

Detoxification—Discontinuation of the use of an illicit drug or a self-administered prescription medication. The process of sobering up and withdrawing from toxic or poisonous effect of alcohol and/or other drugs. The process carried out by the liver in changing chemicals like alcohol into nontoxic substances.

Diabetes mellitus—A disorder in which an inadequate amount of insulin is produced by the pancreas.

Diagnostic assessment instrument—A questionnaire administered for the purpose of obtaining information about medical, psychological, and substance abuse problems.

Diaphoresis—Profuse sweating that is not in response to high temperature or exercise. A common symptom of opiate or sedative-hypnotic withdrawal.

Disulfiram ethanol reaction—The symptoms exhibited as a result of blocking the metabolism of acetaldehyde.

Dopamine—A neurotransmitter that is involved in locomotor activity and the rewarding effects of alcohol and certain drugs of abuse; abnormalities of dopamine regulation may cause depression or psychosis.

Downers—Slang term for drugs that exert a depressant effect on the central nervous system. In general, downers are sedative-hypnotic drugs.

Down-regulation—A decrease in receptor sites caused when excessive numbers of neurotransmitters are available to the receptor over time.

Drug receptors—Specialized areas on the surface of brain cells to which drugs attach and through which they produce their effects.

Dual diagnosis—A diagnosis that includes a concurrent substance use disorder(s) and a psychiatric disorder(s).

Dysphoria—An emotional state characterized by restlessness, anxiety, and depression; an unpleasant mood or a feeling of being ill at ease.

Eczema—A superficial inflammatory process involving the skin.

Edema—Excess accumulation of serous fluid in tissues.

Electroacupuncture—Application of small amounts of electricity to staples or needles at the acupuncture points for opioid withdrawal treatment.

Elimination—The process of removal; the process by which some of the alcohol consumed (2%–5%) is removed from the body via the breath, urine, or sweat glands.

Encephalopathy—Any disease of the essential tissues of the brain.

Endocrine function—The complicated hormonal system that regulates various body processes (e.g., metabolism, growth, temperature, sexual activity, and stress response).

Endorphins—Compounds produced internally that serve as the body's natural opiates. They are more potent than morphine.

Enzyme—A protein that facilitates a chemical reaction but does not itself undergo permanent change.

Epinephrine—A peripheral and central nervous system transmitter; also called adrenaline.

Euphoria—A state of extreme pleasure; the extreme sense of physical and emotional well-being referred to by drug users as the "high."

Family alcoholism—The disease of alcoholism as it affects the whole family system in more than one generation and in all members.

Family intervention—Specific form of intervention involving family members of alcohol and drug addicts designed to benefit the target patient as well as the family constellation.

Family therapy—Treatment of more than one member of a family simultaneously in the same session. The treatment may be supportive, directive, or interpretive.

Gamma-aminobutyric acid (GABA)—A neurotransmitter that inhibits the transfer of an electrical or chemical signal across the synapse of a nerve cell.

Generalized anxiety disorder—A disorder characterized by at least 6 months of persistent and excessive anxiety and worry not resulting from exposure to a drug or medication.

Glutamate—An amino acid that serves as the major excitatory neurotransmitter in the brain.

Grand mal seizure—A type of seizure in which a person falls to the ground unconscious and suffers generalized muscle contractions. The person usually remains unconscious for a time and may have no recall of the episode on awakening. *Petit mal seizures*, by contrast, are characterized by a momentary loss of awareness; an observer may think the person experiencing the seizure is simply daydreaming.

Gynecomastia—The development of mammary glands in the male, sometimes to a functional state.

Half life—Time required by living tissue, an organ, or an organism to eliminate, by biological processes, half the quantity of a substance that has been ingested.

Hallucinogens—A broad group of drugs that cause distortions of sensory perception. The prototype hallucinogen is lysergic acid diethylamide (LSD).

Hangover—The unpleasant physical sensations experienced after the effects of excessive drinking wear off. Symptoms can include nausea, headache, thirst, and fatigue.

Hematocrit—The percentage of red blood cells in whole blood.

Hemorrhagic stroke—Stroke due to rupture of the cerebral blood vessels, often leading to death of the affected brain area.

Hepatic coma—Prolonged unconsciousness that occurs as a consequence of severe liver disease, such as cirrhosis or hepatitis.

Hepatic encephalopathy—A progressive metabolic liver disorder that results in altered intellectual function and emotion, and disturbed psychomotor and behavioral regulation.

Hepatitis—Inflammation of the liver, with accompanying liver cell damage and risk of death. Hepatitis may be of limited duration or a chronic condition. It may be caused by viral infection, as well as chronic exposure to poisons, chemicals, or drugs of abuse, such as alcohol.

Heroin—An illegal opiate drug. Its addictive properties are manifested by the need for persistent, repeated use of the drug (craving) and by the fact that attempts to stop using the drug lead to physical and psychological withdrawal symptoms.

Hippocampus—A region in the temporal lobe of the brain that is thought to play a role in learning and memory as well as in alcohol withdrawal seizures.

Holiday heart syndrome—Cardiac rhythm disturbances following weekend or holiday drinking sprees.

Homeostasis—A tendency of biological systems to maintain stability while continually adjusting to conditions that are optimal for survival.

Hormone—A chemical transmitter substance produced by cells and transported via the bloodstream to cells and organs on which it has specific regulatory effect.

Human Immunodeficiency Virus (HIV)—The infectious virus responsible for acquired immunodeficiency syndrome (AIDS).

Hyperreflexia—An exaggerated response of muscle reflexes which indicates that the nervous system is in an excited state. May occur during withdrawal from sedative-hypnotic agents or alcohol.

Hypersomnolence—Abnormally sleepy or drowsy.

Hypertension—Abnormally high blood pressure. Usually defined as a resting blood pressure greater than 140 mm Hg (systolic) and 90 mm Hg (diastolic).

Hyperthermia—Increased temperature.

Hypnosis—An altered state of awareness in which the individual is extremely responsive to suggestions of the hypnotist.

Hypoglycemia—An abnormally low level of sugar in the blood.

Hypotension—Abnormally low blood pressure.

Hypothalamus—A region of the brain that is involved in basic behavioral and physiological function; regulates water balance, body temperature, sleep, food intake, and the development of secondary sexual characteristics.

Illusion—A mental impression derived from the misinterpretation of sensory stimuli.

Immune response—The production of immunoglobulins, antibodies, lymphocytes, and other substance and cells to defend the body against invading foreign materials or substances.

Immunosuppression—The inability of the body to produce antibodies to fight off infections.

Infarction—Death of an organ or tissue resulting from interruption of its blood supply.

Inhalant—A volatile substance that is introduced into the body via the lungs and readily crosses the blood-brain barrier where it is absorbed by brain tissue.

Injury—A wound, usually as a result of damage applied to the body by an external force.

Instrument—A measurement tool, usually a questionnaire, that is used for gathering information about an individual to aid screening, assessment, diagnosis, and/or clinical decision-making.

Intervention—Process of systematically interceding with an individual who is addicted to alcohol and/or other drugs, with the aim of overcoming denial and assisting the individual to initiate treatment.

Intoxication—An abnormal acute or chronic physiological state that is essentially a poisoning resulting from use of a substance impairing normal function of the nervous system.

Intracerebral stroke—A type of hemorrhagic stroke characterized by bleeding that occurs within the brain tissue.

Ischemic stroke—Impaired flow of blood to the brain resulting from obstruction of a blood vessel, due either to narrowing of the vessel or to an embolism; blockage of cerebral blood vessels, leading to an area of reduced oxygen supply.

Jaundice—Yellowness of skin, sclera, and excretions due to a high amount of bilirubin. It is not a disease, but a symptom of one of a number of different diseases and disorders of the liver, gallbladder, and blood.

Kindling—The property by which a drug will produce certain symptoms only after taking consecutive doses.

Korsakoff's syndrome—An organic brain syndrome associated with prolonged, heavy ingestion of alcohol, characterized by amnesia for recent events, an inability to form new memories, confabulation, and sometimes hallucinations and agitation. *See* Wernicke-Korsakoff syndrome.

Limbic system—Parts of the cerebral cortex, hippocampus, hypothalamus, and other brain structures that together function in the expression of emotional behavior.

Locus ceruleus—Located in the pons; the site of most norepinephrine cell bodies with connections throughout the brain.

Loss of control—An addict's inability to set limits.

Lysergic Acid Diethylamide (LSD)—A hallucinogenic drug derived from fungus that grows on rye or from morning glory seeds.

Malaria—An infectious disease characterized by periodic chills and high fever.

Marijuana—The dried leaves and flowering tops of the Indian hemp plant *cannabis sativa*; also called "pot" and "weed." It can be smoked or prepared in a tea or food.

Medial forebrain bundle—A group of neuron fibers containing dopamine and norepinephrine pathways that project from the midbrain to the forebrain.

Medical comorbidity—Presence of two illness at one time.

Medulla oblongata—The part of the hindbrain that houses the nerve centers for both motor and sensory nerves, where heart rate and respirations are controlled.

Mesolimbic dopamine pathway—A group of dopamine-containing neurons that have their cell bodies in the midbrain and their terminals in the forebrain; believed to be involved in reinforcing behaviors.

Metabolic tolerance—An increase in the breakdown of chemicals as a result of continuous exposure, causing a faster elimination of the chemical from the blood.

Metabolism—The various physical and chemical processes involved in the changing of a substance in the body from an active to an inactive compound.

Midbrain—The part of the brain located just above the pons. It contains nerve pathways between the cerebral hemispheres and the medulla oblongata, and also contains the center for visual reflexes, such as moving the head and eyes.

Misuse—Occurs when alcohol and drugs are sought in order to deal with problems, to get along with others, or to have a good time.

Modality—A specific type of treatment (technique, method, or procedure) that is used to relieve symptoms or induce behavior change. Modalities of alcohol and other drug abuse treatment include, but are not limited to, inpatient social milieu treatment, group therapy, and individual counseling.

Monoamine Oxidase (MAO) inhibitors—A class of antidepressant drugs.

Mood disorders—Depressive and manic disorders.

Morbidity—A state or condition of severe illness or disease.

Motor neuron—A neuron responsible for conveying motor impulses to muscles.

Myocardial infarction—Death of heart tissue resulting from restriction or interruption of blood supply to the heart muscle; a "heart attack."

Myocardium—The heart muscle.

Naltrexone (Trexan)—A long-acting, orally effective drug that inhibits the euphoric effects of narcotics and is used as a maintenance therapy for addicts.

Narcotic—Originally a group of drugs producing effects similar to those of morphine; often used to refer to any substance that sedates and causes a sense of euphoria, has a depressive effect, and/or causes dependence; synonym: opioid.

Needle tracks—Bruising, collapsed veins, or a series of small holes on the surface of the skin caused by chronic injection of drugs into the veins (intravenous injection), or muscle (intramuscular injection), or under the skin (subcutaneous injection).

Neuroadaptation—The process by which the function of the brain cells changes in response to exposure to drugs. These adaptive changes may include increases in the number of receptor sites, alterations in the shape of the receptors, or changes in the chemical function of the cell.

Neuroendocrine—The interactions between the endocrine and nervous systems.

Neuromodulator—A substance that modifies the function or effect of a neurotransmitter.

Neuropathy—Any functional disturbance or pathological change in the peripheral nervous system.

Neurotransmitter—A chemical messenger released by a neuron to excite or inhibit adjacent neurons; a biochemical messenger that helps to transmit signals from one nerve to another in the brain and central nervous system.

Nigrostriatal dopamine pathway—A group of dopamine-containing neurons with their cell bodies located in the substantia nigra of the midbrain and their terminals in the corpus striatum. Deterioration of this pathway is associated with Parkinson's disease.

Nitrites—Class of compounds from nitrous acid that act as potent vasodilators.

Noradrenaline—A neurotransmitter, formed naturally in the body's sympathetic nerve endings and adrenal gland, that controls a number of brain systems and is implicated in mood and anxiety disorders as well as aggressive behavior.

Norepinephrine—A neurotransmitter with various diffuse regulatory functions; important in arousal and learning.

Nucleus—A spherical body in a cell that controls cell growth, metabolism, and reproduction.

Nucleus accumbens—A dopaminergic projection system; also part of the reward center.

Nystagmus—A jerky movement of the eyes. May be seen in persons who are intoxicated as a result of ingestion of alcohol, sedative-hypnotic agents, or phencyclidine.

Omnipotence—Having unlimited power.

Opioids—Any compound from the milky juice of the poppy plant, *Papaver somniferum*, including opium, morphine, codeine, and heroin; a type of depressant drug that diminishes pain and central nervous system activity.

Organic brain syndrome—Any mental disorder caused by or associated with impairment of brain tissue function.

Osteopenia—Any condition involving reduced bone mass.

Osteoporosis—Demineralization of bone; it may be idiopathic or secondary to other diseases.

Oxidation—The process by which the liver converts alcohol into heat and energy and releases carbon dioxide, which is exhaled, and water, which is eliminated as urine.

Pancreatitis—Inflammation of the pancreas. Alcohol abuse is the most common cause of chronic pancreatitis and a principal cause of acute pancreatitis.

Panic disorder—A disorder characterized by sudden, unexpected, and persistent episodes of intense fear, accompanied by a sense of imminent danger and an urge to escape.

Paralysis—Loss or impairment of motor function in part due to a lesion of the neural or muscular mechanism; impairment of sensory function (sensory paralysis). Results from damage to parts of the nervous system. The kind and degree of paralysis depends on whether the damage is to the central nervous system or the peripheral nervous system.

Paranoia—A type of delusion, or a false idea, that is unchanged by reasoned argument or proof to the contrary. Clinical paranoia involves the delusion that people or events are in some way specially related to oneself. Paranoia often occurs during episodes of high-dose chronic stimulant use and may occur during withdrawal from sedative-hypnotics.

Paraplegia—A form of central nervous system paralysis that affects all the muscles of the parts involved; paralysis of the legs and, in some cases, the lower part of the body.

Parasympathetic nervous system—The part of the autonomic nervous system that opposes the effect of the sympathetic nervous system. Generally, it decreases heart rate and dilates blood vessels.

Paresthesia—An abnormal burning, pricking, tickling, or tingling sensation.

Peptic ulcer—An ulceration of the membrane of the esophagus, stomach, or duodenum caused by the action of the acid gastric juice.

Peripheral edema—The abnormal accumulation of fluid in extremities, causing a swollen appearance.

Peripheral nervous system—The part of the nervous system, outside of the central nervous system, including sensory and motor nerves.

Pharmacodynamic tolerance—An increase in the insensitivity of nerve cells to chemicals resulting from continuous exposure.

Phencyclidine (PCP)—A hallucinogenic drug that alters sensation, mood, and consciousness and distorts hearing, touch, smell, taste, and vision.

Phobia—A marked and persistent fear of specific objects or situations.

Platelets—A component of blood important in the clotting process.

Pneumonia—Inflammation of the alveolar spaces of the lung that causes consolidation of lung tissue as the alveoli fill with exudate (a fluid with a high concentration of protein and cellular debris [phlegm]).

Poly-drug abuse—Abuse of two or more mind-altering substances.

Polyneuropathy—A disease involving several nerves.

Postsynaptic neuron—The neuron that receives the neurotransmitter at its receptor site.

Potentiation—If one drug causes a second drug to be metabolized slower than normal, the drug remains in the system longer than it is supposed to and the effects of the drug are greatly magnified.

Problem drinker—A drinker whose behavior causes personal or public harm. This term includes (and is often used as a euphemism for) the alcoholic, particularly in business and industrial programs.

Proprioception—Any sensory nerve endings that give information concerning movement and position of the body.

Protein synthesis—The process that indirectly promotes muscle-tissue development and increases muscle strength.

Protracted abstinence syndrome—The aggregate of signs and symptoms of drug withdrawal. These signs and symptoms may continue for weeks or months after cessation of drug use. (*Also see* Acute Abstinence syndrome.)

Pseudohallucinations—As opposed to hallucinations; unreal images that the person can distinguish as being unreal.

Psychiatric comorbidity—The presence of psychiatric illness in conjunction with a drug addiction; also known as dual diagnosis.

Psychological dependence—A condition resulting from repeated use of a drug in which the individual must continue to take the drug to satisfy a strong emotional need; the need for a drug that results from the continuous or periodic use of that drug. This need can be characterized by mental and/or physical changes in users which make it difficult for them to control or stop their drug use. They believe that they must have the drug to feel good or normal, or to get by.

Psychosis—A mental disorder characterized by hallucination, mood disturbances, and partial or complete withdrawal from reality.

Quadriplegia—Paralysis of all four limbs.

Raphe nucleus—A series of nuclei that extend from the midline of the medulla to the pons, sending fibers to the hypothalamus, the cerebellum, and the cerebral cortex.

Rapid Eye Movement (REM)—The rapid, jerky movements of the eyes which occur during certain stages of the sleep cycle when dreams occur.

Receptors—Specialized areas on the nerve cell adapted to receive neurotransmitters; a protein in the wall of a neuron or other cell that recognizes and binds to neurotransmitters or other chemical messengers.

Recovery—Regaining health; returning to a state in which individuals no longer engage in problematic behavior and are able to accomplish established goals.

Reinforcement—The process by which an effect appears to increase the probability that a particular behavior will recur.

Relapse—A reversion to use of any mind-altering chemical following a period of abstinence.

Reticular Activating System (RAS)—Nerves located in the brain stem involved in wakefullness.

Retrograde amnesia—The inability to remember events that occurred before the trauma or disorder causing the amnesia.

Sedative-hypnotic—A drug that depresses the central nervous system. This class of drugs includes barbiturates and benzodiazepines.

Sensory nerves—Nerves responsible for transmitting messages to the brain from all parts of the body.

Serotonin—A neurotransmitter that affects mood and behavior and the development of tolerance to alcohol; abnormalities in serotonin levels appear to be associated with aggression, impulsivity, anxiety, and eating disorders.

Sickle cell anemia—A genetically determined abnormal shape to the red blood cell, resulting in recurrent attacks of fever and pain in the arms, legs, and abdomen beginning in early childhood. Treatment is symptomatic.

Skin abscesses—A collection of pus formed as a result of bacterial infection.

Slurred speech—A sign of depressant intoxication. Speech may be garbled, mumbled, and slow.

Sobriety—The quality or condition of personal growth as well as abstinence from alcoholic beverages and other drugs of abuse.

Social drinker—A person who drinks occasionally at social functions and whose drinking does not create personal or social problems.

Somatic nervous system—That part of the nervous system which controls voluntary muscular movement.

Somnolence—Sleepiness, drowsiness.

Spider angioma—A star-shaped swelling due to dilation of the blood vessels.

Spinal Cord Injury (SCI)—A lesion of the spinal cord that causes paralysis of certain parts of the body and corresponding loss of sensation in that area.

Status epilepticus—Rapid succession of epileptic (abnormal electrical activity of the brain caused by overstimulation of the nerves cells in the brain) spasms without intervals of consciousness; brain damage may result.

Stimulant—Any chemical that increases the activity of the central nervous system, usually resulting in sharpened reflexes, increased alertness and energy levels, and either sharpened or distorted perceptions depending on the dose and chemical.

Striae—Pinkish or purplish, scarlike lesions, later becoming white, on the breasts, thighs abdomen, and buttocks, associated with pregnancy, obesity, rapid growth during puberty and adolescence, Cushing's syndrome, and topical or prolonged use of corticosteroids. Sometimes referred to as "stretch marks."

Stroke—Any condition leading to partially or completely restricted blood flow to an organ; often used to denote loss of blood flow to the brain or regions of the brain. Strokes are further divided into the categories of hemorrhagic stroke (bleeding within the brain due to ruptured blood vessels) or ischemic stroke (lack of blood due to interrupted flow) and by the area of the brain affected (subarachnoid stroke, intracerebral stroke).

Subcortical—The area of the brain lying beneath the cortex and the principal area where information from the senses is integrated into complex perceptual images.

Substantia nigra—A small area in the midbrain which is the origin of many dopaminergic neurons.

Sympathetic nervous system—The portion of the autonomic nervous system that usually opposes the parasympathetic nervous system. It is sometimes referred to as the "fight or flight" system, and, among other effects, dilates respiratory passages, increases blood flow to vital organs, and decreases gastrointestinal activity.

Symptoms—Subjective changes in mood, feelings, or bodily sensations.

Synergism—The simultaneous action of separate drugs which together have greater total effect than the sum of their individual effects; the potentiating effects are not additive, but are multiplicative.

Tachycardia—Very rapid heart rate, over 100 beats per minute, whether physiological or pathological.

Tachyphylaxis—An accelerated form of tolerance that produces a decrease or loss of reactivity responses following consecutive doses of a drug; a rapid production of immunity to drugs.

Testosterone—One of the male sex hormones, or androgens, that are produced in the testes.

Tetanus—A highly fatal disease caused by a bacteria and characterized by muscle spasms and convulsions; sometimes referred to as lockjaw.

Thalamus—The large structure situated at the base of the cerebrum. It relays impulses and monitors sensory stimuli.

Thiamine—Vitamin B1; essential for growth and required for normal brain functioning.

Thrombotic stroke—Impaired flow of blood to the brain because of formation of a clot in a blood vessel.

Tinnitus—A noise in the ears, such as ringing or buzzing.

Tolerance—Physical tolerance is the body's ability to overcome the usual effects of a drug so that an increased dosage is needed to achieve the same effect as before for the individual. Also, an individual's ability to compensate for the physical and psychological effects of drug use.

Traumatic Brain Injury (TBI)—Refers to damage to the brain caused by external mechanical forces applied to the head. Injury may involve the cranium or the brain, or both. TBI results in impairment of cognitive abilities and/or physical, emotional, and behavioral functioning.

Traumatic injury—Physical injury or tissue damage caused by external force or violence, which may result from assaults or be self-inflicted; can be fatal or nonfatal; may result in temporary, partial, or permanent disability. Traumatic injuries are often classified as penetrating or blunt.

Treatment—The broad range of planned and continuing inpatient, outpatient, and residential services including, but not limited to, diagnostic evaluation; counseling; medical; psychiatric, psychological, and social service care; and occupational services that may be extended to substance abusers and that is geared toward influencing the behavior of an individual to achieve a state of rehabilitation.

Tremors—An involuntary and rhythmic movement in the muscles of parts of the body, most often the hands, feet, jaw, tongue, or head. Tremors may be caused by stimulants such as amphetamines and caffeine, as well as by withdrawal from depressants.

Tuberculosis—An infectious, inflammatory disease that is chronic in nature and commonly affects the lungs, although it may occur in almost any part of the body.

Unsteady gait—Unsteady, crooked, meandering, and uncoordinated walk, typical of alcohol-impaired individuals.

Up-regulation—An increase in the number of receptors on the brain cells that is caused by continuous contact with drugs.

Vasoconstriction—Constriction of blood vessels.

Vasodilation—Dilation of blood vessels.

Vesicle—A tiny sac containing neurotransmitters in the presynaptic neuron.

Wernicke-Korsakoff Syndrome (WKS)—A neurological disorder thought to be caused by thiamine deficiency. WKS is characterized by cognitive impairment in memory (e.g., anterograde amnesia) as well as deficits in abstraction and problem-solving. Wernicke's encephalopathy is an acute condition characterized by general confusion and incoherent speech. It may or may not precede Korsakoff's syndrome, the chronic condition characterized by anterograde amnesia.

Withdrawal syndrome—A cluster of characteristic symptoms and reactions of varying intensity, sometimes fatally severe, which ensue on abrupt cessation or reduction in amount of alcohol and/or other drug for which the body has developed a physical dependence.

REFERENCES

Abrams, D. B., & Niaura, R. S. (1987). Social learning theory. In H. T. Blane & K. E. Leonard (Eds.), *Psychological theories of drinking and alcoholism* (pp. 131–178). New York: Guilford Press.

Adams, P. F., & Benson, V. (1993). Current estimates from national health interview survey, 1991. In *Vital Health Statistics, 1992.* Rockville, MD: National Institutes of Health.

Akers, R. L. (1992). *Drugs, alcohol, and society—Social structure, process and policy.* Belmont, CA: Wadsworth Publishing Company.

Al-Anon Family Group Headquarters, Inc. (1987). *Al-Anon speaks to you, the professional.* [Brochure]. New York: Author.

Al-Anon Family Group Headquarters, Inc. (1991). *Youth and the alcoholic parent.* [Brochure]. New York: Author.

Alexander, C., Morello, S., Gould, J., & Peterson, D. (1993). Preventing severe alcohol withdrawal in the general acute care hospital inpatient. *Perspectives on Addictions Nursing, 4,* 3–6.

Alexander, F., & Duff, R. W. (1988). Social interaction and alcohol use in retirement communities. *Gerontologist, 28,* 632–638.

Alldredge, B. K., Lowenstein, D. H., & Simon, R. P. (1989). Placebo-controlled trial of intravenous disphenylhydantoin for short-term treatment of alcohol withdrawal seizures. *American Journal of Medicine, 87,* 645–648.

Allen, J. P., Eckardt, M. J., & Wallen, J. (1988). Screening for alcoholism: Techniques and issues. *Public Health Reports, 103,* 586–592.

Alling, F. A., Johnson, B. D., & Elmoghazy, E. (1990). Cranial electrostimulation (CES) use in the detoxification of opiate-dependent patients. *Journal of Substance Abuse Treatment, 7,* 173–180.

Altura, B. M., & Altura, B. T. (1990). Alcohol, stroke and the cerebral circulation. *Alcohol Health & Research World, 14,* 322–331.

American Dietetic Association. (1990). Position of the American Dietetic Association: Nutrition intervention in treatment and recovery from chemical dependency. *Journal of the American Dietetic Association, 90,* 1274–1276.

American Medical Association (AMA). (1995). *Alcoholism in the elderly: Diagnosis, treatment, and prevention; Guidelines for primary care physicians.* Chicago, IL: Author.

Annegers, J. F., Grabow, J. D., Kurland, L. T., & Laws, E. R. Jr. (1980). The incidence, causes, and secular trends of head trauma in Olmstead County, Minnesota, 1935–1974. *Neurology, 30,* 912–919.

Anton, R. F. (1994). Medications for treating alcoholism. *Alcohol Health & Research World, 18*, 265–271.

Antti-Poika, I. (1986). The assessment of alcohol abuse among injured patients. *Injury, 17*, 359–761.

Antti-Poika, I., Karaharju, E., Roine, R., & Salaspuro, M. (1988). Intervention of heavy drinking—A prospective and controlled study of 438 consecutive injured male patients. *Alcohol & Alcoholism, 23*, 115–121.

Arria, A. M., Tarter, R. E., & Van Thiel, D. H. (1990). Liver-brain relations in alcoholics. *Alcohol Health & Research World, 14*, 112–117.

Ashton, H. (1991). Protracted withdrawal syndromes from benzodiazepines. *Journal of Substance Abuse Treatment, 8*, 19–28.

Atkinson, R. M., Tolson. R. L., & Turner, J. A. (1990). Late versus early onset problem drinking in older men. *Alcoholism: Clinical and Experimental Research, 14*, 574–579.

Azrin, N. H., Sisson, R. W., Meyers, R., & Godley, M. (1982). Alcoholism treatment by disulfiram and community reinforcement therapy. *Journal of Behavior Therapy and Experimental Psychiatry, 13*, 105–112.

Babor, T. F., & Grant, M. (1989). From clinical research to secondary prevention: International collaboration in the development of the alcohol use disorders identification test (AUDIT). *Alcohol Health & Research World, 13*, 371–374.

Bagasra, O., Kajdacey-Balla, A., & Lischner, H. W. (1989). Effects of alcohol ingestion on in vitro susceptibility of peripheral blood mononucleur cells to infection with HIV and of selected T-cell functions. *Alcoholism: Clinical and Experimental Research, 13*, 636–643.

Baker, S. P., O'Neill, B., Ginsburg, M. J., & Li, G. (1992). *The injury fact book* (2nd ed.). New York: Oxford University Press.

Ballenger, J. C., & Post. R. M. (1978). Kindling as a model for alcohol withdrawal syndromes. *British Journal of Psychiatry, 133*, 1–14.

Bean-Bayog, M. (1986). Psychopathology produced by alcoholism. In R. E. Meyer (Ed.), *Psychopathology and addictive disorders*. New York: Guilford.

Beasley, J. (1995). Alcohol, drug addiction recovery rate can be doubled with program of nutritional support. *Health News & Review, 4*, 1–3.

Beasley, J., & Knightly, S. (1994). *Food for recovery*. New York: Crown.

Becker, V., Tonnesen, H., Kaas-Claesson, N., & Gluud, C. (1989). Menstrual disturbances and fertility in chronic alcoholic women. *Drug and Alcohol Dependence, 24*, 75–82.

Beeder, A. B., & Millman, R. B. (1992). Treatment of patient with psychopathology and substance abuse. In J. Lowinson, P. Ruiz, & R. Millman (Eds.), *Substance abuse: A comprehensive text* (2nd ed., pp. 675–690). Baltimore: Williams & Wilkins.

Bjorneboe, A.-E. A. et al. (1988). Calcium status and calcium-regulating hormones in alcoholics. *Alcoholism: Clinical and Experimental Research, 12*, 229–232.

Bohn, M. J., Babor, T. F., & Kranzler, H. R. (1995). The alcohol use disorders identification test (AUDIT): Validation of a screening instrument for use in medical settings. *Journal of Studies on Alcohol, 56*, 423–432.

Bradley, K. A. (1992). Management of alcoholism in the primary care setting. *Western Journal of Medicine, 156*, 273–277.

Brown, M. E., Anton, R. F., Malcolm, R., & Ballenger, J. C. (1988). Alcohol detoxification and withdrawal seizures: Clinical support for a kindling hypothesis. *Biological Psychiatry, 23*, 507–514.

Brown, S. (1985). *Treating the alcoholic: A developmental model of recovery.* New York: John Wiley & Sons.

Brown, S. (1994). Alcoholism and trauma: A theoretical overview and comparison. *Journal of Psychoactive Drugs, 26*, 345–355.

Bruno, F. (1989). Buspirone in the treatment of alcoholic patients. *Psychopathology, 22*(Suppl. 1), 49–59.

Bufe, C. (1991). *Alcoholics anonymous: Cult or cure.* Tuscon, AZ: See Sharp Press.

Bullock, M. L., Culliton, P. D., & Olander, R. T. (1989). Controlled trial of acupuncture for severe recidivist alcoholism. *Lancet, 1*, 1435–1439.

Buss, A., & Cramer, C. (1989). *Incidence of alcohol use by people with disabilities: A Wisconsin survey of persons with a disability.* Madison, WI: Office of Persons with Disabilities.

Butters, N., & Cermak, L. S. (1980). *Alcoholic Korsakoff's syndrome: An information-processing approach to amnesia.* New York: Academic Press.

Caracci, G., & Miller, N. S. (1991). Epidemiology and diagnosis of alcoholism in the elderly. *International Journal of Geriatric Psychiatry, 6*, 511–515.

Cataldo, C. B., Debruyne, L. K., & Whitney, E. N. (1992). *Nutrition and diet therapy* (pp. 99–150). New York: West Publishing Company.

Center for Substance Abuse Research (CSAT). (1995, July 3). More than 13 million adult Americans have an alcohol problem: Highest rates found among young adults [1 paragraph]. *CESAR FAX* [Fax], *4*(26). (Available by Voice: 301-403-8329; Fax: 301-403-8342; E-mail: CESAR@cesar.umd.edu)

Cesare, J., Morgan, A. S., Felice, P. R., & Edge, V. (1990). Characteristics of blunt and personal violent injuries. *Journal of Trauma, 30*, 176–182.

Charness, M. E. (1990). Alcohol and the brain. *Alcohol Health & Research World, 14*, 85–89.

Charness, M. E., Simon, R. P., & Greenberg, D. A. (1989). Ethanol and the nervous system. *New England Journal of Medicine, 321*, 442–454.

Clark, D. E., McCarthy, E., & Robinson, E. (1985). Trauma as a symptom of alcoholism. *Annuals of Emergency Medicine, 14*, 274.

Clark, H. W., Sees, K. L., & Nathan, J. A. (1988). Clinical and legal aspects of nonphysician prescription of vitamins, amino acids, and other nutritional supplements. *Journal of Psychoactive Drugs, 20,* 355–374.

Clark, R. F., & Harchelroad, F. (1991). Toxicology screening of the trauma patient: A changing profile. *Annals of Emergency Medicine, 20,* 151–153.

Cohen, S. (1988). *The chemical brain—The neurochemistry of addictive disorders.* Minneapolis, MN: CompCare Publishers.

Colsher, P. L., & Wallace, R. B. (1990). Elderly men with histories of heavy drinking: Correlates and consequences. *Journal of Studies on Alcohol, 6,* 528–535.

Combs-Orme, T., Taylor, J. R., Scott, E. B., & Holmes, S. J. (1983). Violent deaths among alcoholics: A descriptive study. *Journal of Studies on Alcohol, 44,* 938–949.

Cook, B. L., Winokur, G., Garvey, M. J., & Beach, V. (1991). Depression and previous alcoholism in the elderly. *British Journal of Psychiatry, 158,* 72–75.

Cooney, N. L., Baker, L. H., & Ponerleau, O. F. (1983). Cue exposure for relapse prevention in alcohol treatment. In K. D. Craig & R. J. McMahon (Eds.), *Advances in clinical behavior therapy* (pp. 194–210). New York: Brunner/Mazel.

Cooper, M. L. (1992). Alcohol and increased behavioral risk for AIDS. *Alcohol Health & Research World, 16,* 64–72.

Council on Mental Health. (1971). Narcotics and medical practice. *Journal of the American Medical Association, 218,* 578–583.

Council on Scientific Affairs. (1996). Alcoholism in the elderly. *Journal of the American Medical Association, 275,* 1–6.

Crist, D. A., & Milby, J. B. (1990). Psychometric and neuropsychological assessment. In W. D. Lerner & M. A. Barr (Eds.), *Handbook of hospital based substance abuse treatment.* New York: Pergamon Press.

Crowe, A. H., & Reeves, R. (1994). *Treatment for alcohol and other drug abuse—Opportunities for coordination.* (Technical Assistance Publication (TAP) Series 11, DHHS Publication No. SMA 94-2075). Rockville, MD: U.S. Department of Health and Human Services.

Cutler, S. F., Wallace, P. G., & Haines, A. P. (1988). Assessing alcohol consumption in general practice patients—A comparison between questionnaire and interview. *Alcohol, 23,* 441–450.

Cutting, J. (1978). The relationship between Korsakoff's syndrome and "alcoholic dementia." *British Journal of Psychiatry, 132,* 240–251.

Dackis, C. A., & Gold, M. S. (1992). Psychiatric hospitals for treatment of dual diagnosis. In J. H. Lowinson, P. Ruiz, R. B. Millman, & J.G. Langrod (Eds.), *Substance abuse: A comprehensive textbook* (2nd ed., pp. 467–485). Baltimore: Williams & Wilkins.

Davis–Cox, M. I., Fletcher, T. L., Turner, J. N., Szarwoski, D., & Shain, W. (1996). Three day exposure to low-dose ethanol alters guanine nucleotide binding protein expression in the developing rat

hippocampus. *Journal of Pharmacology and Experimental Therapeutics, 276,* 758–764.
Dean, J. C., & Poremba, G. A. (1983). The alcoholic stigma and the disease concept. *International Journal on Addictions, 18,* 739–751.
Department of Justice. (1994). Code of federal regulations (28 CFR Part 36) [Section 36.104 Subpart 4—General Definitions] pg. 469 Part 36 Nondiscrimination on the basis of disability by public accommodations and in commercial facilities. Washington, DC: Author.
de Miranda, J., & Cherry, L. (1989). California responds: Changing treatment systems through advocacy for the disabled. *Alcohol Health & Research, 13,* 154–157.
DeSoto, C. B., O'Donnell, W. E., & DeSoto, J. L. (1989). Long-term recovery in alcoholics. *Alcoholism: Clinical and Experimental Research, 13,* 693–697.
Dietz, P. E., & Baker, S. P. (1974). Drowning: Epidemiology and prevention. *American Journal of Public Health, 64,* 303–312.
Dorian, P., Sellers, E. M., Reed, K. L., Warsh, J. J., Hamilton, C., Kaplan, H. L., & Fan, T. (1983). Amitriptyline and ethanol: Pharmacokinetic and pharmacodynamic interaction. *European Jounal of Clinical Pharmacology, 25,* 325–331.
Doweiko, H. E. (1993). *Concepts of chemical dependency* (2nd ed.). Pacific Grove, CA: Brooks/Cole Publishing Company.
Dufour, M. S., Archer, L., & Gordis, E. (1992). Alcohol and the elderly. *Clinics in Geriatric Medicine, 8,* 127–141.
Dyken, M. L., Wolf, P. A., Barnett, H. J. M., Bergan, J. J., Hass, W. K., Kannel, W. B., Kuller, L., Kurtzke, J. F., Sundt. T. M. (1984). Risk factors in stroke: A statement for physicians by the subcommittee on risk factors and stroke of the stroke council. *Stroke, 15,* 1105–1111.
Egbert, A. M. (1993). The older alcoholic: Recognizing the subtle clinical clues. *Geriatrics, 48,* 7.
el-Guebaly, N., & el-Guebaly, A. (1981). Alcohol abuse in ancient Egypt: The recorded evidence. *International Journal of the Addictions, 16,* 1207–1221.
Ellis, A., & McClure, J. (1992). Inpatient treatment of alcohol problems—predicting and preventing relapse. *Alcohol & Alcoholism, 27,* 449–456.
Ewing, J. A. (1984). Detecting alcoholism: The CAGE questionnaire. *Journal of the Amercian Medical Association, 252,* 1905–1907.
Ewing, J. A., & Rouse, B. A. (1970, February 3). *Identifying the hidden alcoholic.* Paper presented at the Twenty-Ninth International Congress on Alcohol and Drug Dependence, Sydney, Australia.
Fassoulaki, A., Farinotti, R., Servin, F., & Desmonts, J. M. (1993). Chronic alcoholism increases the induction dose of propofol in humans. *Anesthesia and Analgesia, 77,* 553–556.
Fawcett, J., Clark, D. C., Gibbonds, R. D., Aagesen, C. A., Pisani, V. D., Tilkin, J. M., Sellers, D., & Stutzman, D. (1984). Evaluation of

lithium therapy for alcoholism. *Journal of Clinical Psychiatry, 45*, 494–499.

Feinman, L. (1989). Absorption and utilization of nutrients in alcoholism. *Alcohol Health & Research World, 13*, 207–210.

Fell, J. C. (1992, March 23–25). *Alcohol-related traffic injuries: What do we know? What do we need?* Paper presented at the Secretary's National Conference on Alcohol-Related Injuries, U S. Department of Health and Human Services, Washington, DC.

Finlayson, R. E., Hurt, R. D., Davis, L. J., & Morse, R. M. (1988). Alcoholism in elderly persons: A study of the psychiatric and psychosocial features of 216 inpatients. *Mayo Clinic Proceedings, 63*, 761–768.

Finnegan, L. P., & Kandall, S. R. (1992). Maternal and neonatal effects of alcohol and drugs. In J. H. Lowinson, P. Ruiz, & R. S. Millman (Eds.), *Substance abuse: A comprehensive textbook*. Baltimore, MD: Williams & Wilkens.

Fleming, M. F., & Barry, K. L. (1992). *Addictive disorders*. St. Louis: Mosby-Year Book.

French, S. W. (1991). The mechanism of organ injury in alcoholics: Implications for therapy. *Alcohol & Alcoholism*, (Suppl. 1), 57–63.

Friedman, H. A. (1990). Alcohol and hypertension. *Alcohol Health & Research World, 14*, 313–319.

Friedman, H. A. (1992). Alcohol, arrhythmia, and sudden death. *Alcohol Health & Research World, 16*, 87–91.

Fuller, R. K., Branchey, L., Brightwell, D. R., Derman, R. M., Emrick, C. D., Iber, R. K., James, K. E., Lacoursiere, R. B., Lee, K. K., Lowenstam, I., Maany, I., Neiderhiser, D., Nocks, J. J., & Shaw, S. (1986). Disulfiram treatment of alcoholism: A Veterans Administration cooperative study. *Journal of the American Medical Association, 256*, 1449–1455.

Galanter, M., Egelko, S., & Edwards, H. (1993). Rational recovery: Alternative to AA for addiction? *Amercian Journal of Drug and Alcohol Abuse, 19*, 499–510.

Garro, A. J., Espina, N., & Lieber, C. S. (1992). Alcohol and cancer. *Alcohol Health & Research World, 16*, 81–86.

Gavaler, J. S. (1988). Effects of moderate consumption of alcoholic beverages on endocrine function in postmenopausal women: Bases for hypothesis. In M. Galanter (Ed.), *Recent developments in alcoholism* (Vol. 6, pp. 229–251). New York: Plenum Press.

Gentilello, L. M., Donovan, D. M., Dunn, C. W., & Rivara, F. P. (1995). Alcohol interventions in trauma centers: Current practice and future decision. *Journal of the American Medical Association, 274*, 1043–1048.

Girre, C., Facy, F., Lagier, G., & Dally, S. (1988). Detection of blood benzodiazepines in injured people. Relationship with alcoholism. *Drug and Alcohol Dependence, 21*, 61–65.

Glaze, L. W., & Coggan, P. G. (1987). Efficacy of an alcoholism self-report questionnaire in a residency clinic. *Journal of Family Practice, 25*, 60–41.

Gleick, E. (1995, July 10). Sobering times for AA. *Time*, 49–50.

Gluckman, S. J., Dvorak, V. C., & MacGregor, R. R. (1977). Host defenses during prolonged alcohol consumption in a controlled environment. *Archives of Internal Medicine, 137*, 1539–1543.

Gold, M. S. (1992). Cocaine (and crack): Clinical aspects. In J. Lowinson, P. Ruiz, & R. Millman (Eds.), *Substance abuse: A comprehensive textbook* (2nd ed., pp. 205–221). Baltimore: Williams & Wilkins.

Gomberg, E. (1990). Drugs, alcohol, and aging. In L. T. Kozlowski, H. M. Annis, H. D. Cappell, F. B. Glaser, M. S. Goodstadt, Y. Israel, H. Kalant, E. M. Sellers, & E. R. Vingilis (Eds.), *Research advances in alcohol and drug problems* (Vol. 10, pp. 171–213). New York: Plenum Press.

Goodman, L. (1988, August). Would your assessment spot a hidden alcoholic? *RN, 51*, 56–60.

Gorelick, P. B. (1989). The status of alcohol as a risk factor for stroke. *Stroke, 20*, 1607–1610.

Gorelick, P. B. (1990). Stroke from alcohol and drug abuse: A current social peril. *Postgraduate Medicine, 88*, 171–178.

Gorelick, P. B., & Kelly, M. A. (1992). Alcohol as a risk factor for stroke. *Heart Disease and Stroke, 1*, 255–258.

Graham, K. (1986). Identifying and measuring alcohol abuse among the elderly: Serious problems with existing instrumentation. *Journal on Studies of Alcoholism, 47*, 322–326.

Grant, B. F., Dufour, M. S., & Harford, T. C. (1988). Epidemiology of alcoholic liver disease. *Seminars in Liver Disease, 8*, 12–25.

Greenspan, K., & Smith, T. J. (1991). Perspectives on alcohol and medication interactions. *Journal of Alcohol and Drug Education, 36*, 103–107.

Greenstein, R. A., Fudala, P. J., & O'Brien, C. P. (1992). Alternative pharmacotherapies for opiate addiction. In J. H. Lowinson, P. Ruiz, R. B. Millman, & J. G. Langrod (Eds.), *Substance abuse: A comprehensive textbook* (2nd ed.). Baltimore: Williams & Wilkins.

Guthrie, S. K. (1989). The treatment of alcohol withdrawal. *Pharmacotherapy, 9*, 131–143.

Guram, M. S., Howden, C. W., & Holt, S. (1992). Alcohol and drug interactions. *Practical Gastroenterology, 16*, 50–54.

Gurion, J. (1990, March). Remaking our lives. *American Health*, 50–52.

Harrington, C. R., Putnam, S. L., Waters, W. J., & Colt, A. M. (1989). The community gatekeeper training model for reducing alcohol abuse and alcohol-related injury. *Rhode Island Medical Journal, 72*, 459–463.

Heinemann, A. W. (1991). Substance abuse and spinal cord injury. *Paraplegia News, 45*, 16–19.

Heinemann, A. W., Doll, M., & Schnoll, S. (1989). Treatment of alcohol abuse in people with recent spinal cord injuries. *Alcohol Health and Research World, 13*, 110–117.

Heinemann, A. W., Keen, M., Donohue, R., & Schnoll, S. (1988). Alcohol use by persons with recent spinal cord injury. *Archives of Physical Medicine and Rehabilitation, 69*, 619–624.

Hester, R. K., & Miller, W. R. (1989). Self-control training. In R. K. Hester & W. R. Miller (Eds.), *Handbook of alcoholism treatment approaches: Effective alternatives* (pp. 141–149). New York: Pergamon Press.

Hingson, R., & Howland, J. (1987). Alcohol as a risk factor for injury or death resulting from accidental falls: A review of the literature. *Journal of Studies on Alcohol, 48*, 212–219.

Hinmichsen, J. J. (1990). Alcoholics Anonymous: The heart of treatment for alcoholism. *Aging, 361*, 13–17.

Hofmann, F. G. (1983). *A handbook on drugs and alcohol abuse* (2nd ed., pp. 96–116). New York: Oxford University Press.

Holder, H. (1992). *Effects of alcohol, alone and in combination with medications.* Walnut Creek, CA: Prevention Research Center.

Horn, J. L., Skinner, H. A., Wanberg, K., & Foster, F. M. (1984). *The alcohol use questionnaire (ADS).* Toronto, Canada: Drug Addiction Research Foundation.

Hoshino, J. (1992). Assessment of adolescent substance abuse. In G. W. Lawson & A. W. Lawson (Eds.), *Adolescent substance abuse: Etiology, treatment and prevention.* Gaithersburg, MD: Aspen Publishers.

Howland, J., & Hingson, R. (1987). Alcohol as a risk factor for injuries or death due to fires and burns: Review of the literature. *Public Health Reports, 102*, 475–483.

Institute of Medicine. (1990a). *Broadening the base of treatment for alcohol problems.* Washington, DC: National Academy Press.

Institute of Medicine. (1990b). Effectiveness of treatment. In D. R. Gerstein & H. J. Harwood (Eds.), *Treating drug problems* (Vol. 1, pp. 11–21). Washington, DC: National Academy Press.

Isaacson, J. H., Butler, R., Zacharedk, M., & Tzelepis, A. (1994). Screening with the alcohol use disorders identification test (AUDIT) in an inner-city population. *Journal of General Internal Medicine, 9*, 550–553.

Ishii, H., Takagi, T., Okuno, F., Ebihara, Y., Tashireo, M., & Tsuchiya, M. (1983). Halothane-induced hepatic necrosis in ethanol-pretreated rats. In C. S. Lieber (Ed.), *Biological approaches to alcoholism* (National Institute on Alcohol Abuse and Alcoholism Research Monograph No. 11, DHHS Publication No. ADM 83-1261, pp. 152–157). Washington, DC: U.S. Government Printing Office.

Jacobson, J. M. (1992). Alcoholism and tuberculosis. *Alcohol Health & Research World, 16*, 39–45.

Jernigan, T. L., & Ostergaard, A. L. (1995). When alcoholism affects memory functions. *Alcohol Health & Research World, 19*, 104–107.

Kadden, R., Carroll, K., Donovan, D., Cooney, N., Monti, P., Abrams, D., Litt, M., & Hester, R. (Eds.). (1992). *Cognitive-behavioral coping skills therapy manual.* Rockville, MD: National Institute on Alcohol Abuse and Alcoholism.

Katims, J. J., Ng, L. K. Y., & Lowinson, J. H. (1992). Acupuncture and transcutaneous electrical nerve stimulation: Afferent nerve stimulation (ANS) in the treatment of addiction. In J. H. Lowinson, P. Ruiz, R. B. Millman, & J. G. Langrod (Eds.), *Substance abuse: A comprehensive textbook* (2nd ed.). Baltimore: Williams & Wilkins.

Keso, L., Kivisaari, A., & Salaspuro, M. (1988). Fractures on chest radiographs in detection of alcoholism. *Alcohol and Alcoholism, 23,* 53–56.

Kinney, J., & Leaton, G. (1991). *Loosening the grip—A handbook of alcohol information* (4th ed.). St. Louis, MO: Mosby-Year Book.

Kissin, B. (1974). Interactions ethyl alcohol and other drugs. In B. Kissin & H. Befleiter (Eds.), *The biology of alcoholism: Vol. 3. Clinical pathology* (pp. 109–162). New York: Plenum Press.

Klatsky, A. L. (1990). Alcohol and coronary artery disease. *Alcohol Health & Research World, 14,* 289–300.

Kleber, H. D. (1994). *Assessment and treatment of cocaine-abusing methadone-maintained patients* (Treatment Improvement Protocol [TIPS] Series 10, DHHS Publication No. SMA 94-3003). Rockville, MD: U.S. Department of Health and Human Services.

Klein, S., & Iber, F. L. (1991). Alcoholism and associated malnutrition in the elderly. *Nutrition, 7,* 75–79.

Klemm, W. R. (1979). Effects of ethanol on nerve impulse activity. In E. Majchrowicz & E. P. Noble (Eds.), *Biochemistry and pharmacology of ethanol* (Vol. 2, pp. 243–267). New York: Plenum Press.

Korsten, M. A. (1989). Alcoholism and pancreatitis: Does nutrition play a role? *Alcohol Health & Research World, 13,* 232–237.

Kosten, T. R., Rounsanville, B. J., & Kleber, H. D. (1987). A 2.5 year follow-up of cocaine use among treated opiate addicts. *Archives of General Psychiatry, 44,* 281–284.

Kraus, J. S. (1992). Delivery of substance abuse services during spinal cord injury rehabilitation. *Journal of Neurorehabilitation, 2,* 45–51.

Krista, A. (1986). *The book of stress survival* (pp. 133–145). New York: Simon & Schuster.

Kruger, T. E., & Jerrells, T. R. (1992). Potential role of alcohol in human immunodeficiency virus infection. *Alcohol Health & Research World, 16,* 57–63.

Krupp, N. E. (1968). Psychiatric implications of chronic and crippling illness. *Psychosomatics, 9,* 109–113.

Lands, W. E. M., & Zakhari, A. (1990). Alcohol and cardiovascular disease. *Alcohol Health & Research World, 14,* 304–312.

Langlais, P. J. (1995). Alcohol-related thiamine deficiency—Impact on cognitive and memory functioning. *Alcohol Health & Research World, 19,* 113–121.

Langley, M. J. (1991). Preventing post-injury alcohol-related problems: A behavioral approach. In B. T. McMahon & L. R. Shaw (Eds.), *Work worth doing: Advances in brain injury rehabilitation.* Orlando: Paul M. Deutsch Press.

Larson, J. M. (1994). *Seven weeks to sobriety: The proven progress to fight alcoholism through nutrition.* New York: Random House.

Lehman, L. B., Pilich, A., & Andrews, N. (1993, Fall). Neurological disorders resulting from alcoholism. *Alcohol Health and Research World,* 305–310.

Leo, M. A., & Lieber, C. S. (1989). Alcohol and vitamin A. *Alcohol Health & Research World, 13,* 250–254.

Lieber, C. S. (1976). The metabolism of alcohol. *Scientific American, 234,* 3–11.

Lieber, C. S. (1988). The influence of alcohol on nutritional status. *Nutrition Reviews, 46,* 241–254.

Lieber, C. S. (1989). Alcohol and nutrition: An overview. *Alcohol Health & Research World, 13,* 197–205.

Lieber, C. S. (1992). Interaction of ethanol with other drugs. In C. S. Lieber (Ed.), *Medical and nutritional complications of alcoholism: Mechanisms and management* (pp. 165–183). New York: Plenum Press.

Lieber, C. S., Garro, A. J., Leo, M. A., & Worner, T. M. (1986). Mechanisms for the interrelationship between alcohol and cancer. *Alcohol Health & Research World, 10,* 10–17, 40–50.

Linnoila, M., Mattila, M. J., & Kitchell, B. S. (1979). Drug interactions with alcohol. *Drugs, 18,* 299–311.

Lishman, W. A. (1986). Alcoholic dementia: A hypothesis. *Lancet, 1,* 1184–1186.

Liskow, B. I., & Goodwin, D. W. (1987). Pharmacological treatment of alcohol intoxication, withdrawal, and dependence: A critical review. *Journal of Studies on Alcohol, 48,* 356–370.

Lloyd, C. W., & Williams, R. H. (1948). Endocrine changes associated with Laennec's cirrhosis of the liver. *American Journal of Medicine, 4,* 315–330.

Lowenfels, A. B., & Miller, T. T. (1984). Alcohol and trauma. *Annals of Emergency Medicine, 13,* 1056–1060.

Lowenstein, S. R., Weissberg, M. P., & Terry, D. (1990). Alcohol intoxication, injuries, and dangerous behaviors—And the revolving emergency department door. *Journal of Trauma, 30,* 1252–1258.

Luckmann, J., & Sorensen, K. C. (1974). *Medical-surgical nursing—A psychophysiologic approach.* Philadelphia: W.B. Saunders Company.

MacGregor, R. R. (1986). Alcohol and immune defense. *Journal of the American Medical Association, 256,* 1474–1479.

Maisto, S. A., & Connors, G. J. (1990). Clinical diagnostic techniques and assessment tools in alcohol research. *Alcohol Health & Research World, 14,* 232–238.

Malec, E., Malec, T., Gagné, M. A., & Donigier, M. (1996). Buspirone in the treatment of alcohol dependence: A placebo-controlled trial. *Alcoholism: Clinical and Experimental Research, 20*, 307–312.

Manhem, P., Nilsson, L. H., Moberg, A., Wadstein, J., & Hokfelt, B. (1985). Alcohol withdrawal: Effects of clonidine treatment on sympathetic activity, the renin-aldosterone system, and clinical symptoms. *Alcoholism: Clinical and Experimental Research, 9*, 238–243.

Mansfield, G. J., & Cunningham, C. L. (1980). Conditioning and extinction of tolerance to the hypothermic effect of ethanol in rats. *Journal of Comparative and Physiological Psychology, 94*, 962–969.

Marlatt, G. A., & Gordon, J. R. (Eds.). (1985). *Relapse prevention.* New York: Guilford Press.

Mattox, M. (1986). *The nurse's role in recognizing chemical dependency.* Center City, MN: Hazeldon Foundation.

Maull, K. I. (1982). Alcohol abuse: Its implications in trauma care. *Southern Medical Journal, 75*, 794–798.

Maull, K., Clapp, A., & Ellis, L. (1986, February). *Non-vehicular trauma and driver behavior: A comparative study of alcohol-impaired and non-impaired subjects.* Paper presented at the International Congress and Exposition on Alcohol, Accidents, and Injuries, Detroit, MI.

Mayfield, D., McLeod, G., & Hall, P. (1974). The CAGE questionnaire: Validation of a new alcoholism screening instrument. *American Journal of Psychiatry, 131*, 1121–1123.

McCaffery, M. (1988). When your patient is a drug abuser. *Nursing 88, 18*, 49.

McClain, C. J., Van Thiel, D. H., Parker, S., Badzin, L. K., & Gilbert, H. (1979). Alterations in zinc, vitamin A, and retinol-binding protein in chronic alcoholics: A possible mechanism for night blindness and hypogonadism. *Alcoholism: Clinical and Experimental Research, 3*, 135–140.

McCrady, B. S., Noel, N. E., Abrans, D. B., Stout, R. L., Nelson, H. F., & Hay, W. M. (1986). Comparative effectiveness of three types of spouse involvement in outpatient behavioral alcoholism treatment. *Journal of Studies on Alcohol, 47*, 459–467.

McGovern, M. P., & Morrison, D. H. (1992). The chemical use, abuse, and dependence scale (CUAD)—Rationale, reliability, and validity. *Journal of Substance Abuse Treatment, 9*, 27–38.

McLellan, T., & Dembo, R. (1992). *Screening and assessment of alcohol and other drug (AOD) abusing adolescents* (Treatment Improvement Protocol [TIP] Series 3, DHHS Publication No. SMA 93-2009). Rockville, MD: U.S. Department of Health and Human Services.

Melchoir, C. L., & Tavakoff, B. (1981). Modification of environmentally-cued tolerance to ethanol in mice. *Journal of Pharmacology and Experimental Therapeutics, 219*, 175–180.

Merry, J., Reynolds, C. M., Bailey, J., & Coppen, A. (1976). Prophylactic treatment of alcoholism by lithium carbonate: A controlled study. *Lancet*, 481–482.

Messerli, F. H. (Ed.). (1993). *Cardiovascular disease in the elderly* (3rd ed.). Norwell, MA: Kluwer Academic Publishers.

Meyer, R. E. (1986). How to understand the relationship between psychopathology and addictive disorders: Another example of the chicken and the egg. In R. E. Meyer (Ed.), *Psychopathology and addictive disorders* (pp. 3–16). New York, NY: Guilford Press.

Meyers, H. B., Zepeda, S. G., & Murdock, M. A. (1990). Alcohol and trauma—An endemic syndrome. *Western Journal of Medicine, 153*, 149–153.

Miles, M. R. (1995). Alcohol's effect on gene expression. *Alcohol Health & Research World, 19*, 237–243.

Miller, N. S., & Gold, M. S. (1989). Identification and treatment of benzodiazepine abuse. *American Family Physician, 40*, 175–183.

Miller, N. S., & Gold, M. S. (1991). *Alcohol*. New York: Plenum Medical Book Co.

Miller, W. R. (1992). The effectiveness of treatment for substance abuse: Reasons for optimism. *Journal of Substance Abuse Treatment, 9*, 93–102.

Miller, W. R., & Rollnick, S. (1991). *Motivational interviewing: Preparing people to change addictive behavior*. New York: Guilford Press.

Millman, R. B. (1988). Evaluation and clinical management of cocaine abusers. *Journal of Clinical Psychiatry, 49*(Suppl.), 27–33.

Mishkin, G., & Sparadeo, F. R. (1991). *Effects of substance use on recovery from TBI*. Paper presented at the annual meeting of the National Head Injury Foundation, Los Angeles, CA.

Moore, D. (1990). *Research in substance abuse and disabilities: The implications for prevention and treatment*. Paper presented at the National Prevention Research Conference: People With Disabilities, Phoenix, AZ.

Moore, D., & Ford, J. A. (1991). Prevention of substance abuse among persons with disabilities: A demonstration model. *Prevention Forum, 2*, 2.

Moore, D., & Polsgrove, L. (1991). Disabilities, developmental handicaps, and substance misuses: A review. *The International Journal on the Addictions, 26*, 118–123.

Moore, D., & Seigel, H. (1989). Double trouble: Alcohol and other drug use among orthopedically impaired college students. *Alcohol Health & Research World, 13*, 118–123.

Moos, R. H., Finney, J. W., & Cronkite, R. C. (1990). *Alcohol treatment*. New York: Oxford University Press.

Morse, R. M., & Flavin, D. K. (1992). The definition of alcoholism. *Journal of the American Medical Association, 268*, 1012–1014.

Mourer, S. (1992). Understanding substance use in SCI. *SCI Psychosocial Process, 5*, 109–110.

Mufti, S. I., Darban, H. R., & Watson, R. R. (1989). Alcohol, cancer, and immunomodulation. *Critical Reviews in Oncology/Hematology, 9*, 243–261.
Mutchnick, M. G., & Lee, H. H. (1988). Impaired lymphocyte proliferative response to mitogen in alcoholic patients: Absence of a relation to liver disease activity. *Alcoholism: Clinical and Experimental Research, 12*, 155–158.
Naegle, M. (Ed.). (1993). *Substance abuse education in nursing—Volume 3: Curriculum modules*. New York: National League for Nursing Press.
Nair, M. P. N., Schwartz, S. A., Kronfol, Z. A., Heimer, E. P., Pottathil, R., & Greden, J. F. (1990). Immunoregulatory effects of alcohol on lymphocyte responses to human immunodeficiency virus proteins. *Progress in Clinical and Biological Research, 325*, 221–230.
Naranjo, C. A., & Sellers, E. M. (1986). Clinical assessment and pharmacotherapy of the alcohol withdrawal syndrome. In M. Galanter (Ed.), *Recent developments in alcoholism* (Vol. 4, pp. 265–281). New York: Plenum Press.
National Academy of Sciences. (1985). *Injury in America: A continuing public health problem*. Washington, DC: National Academy Press.
National Center for Injury Prevention and Control. (1991). *Ten leading causes of injury death in the United States*. Atlanta, GA: Centers for Disease Control and Prevention.
National Institute on Alcohol Abuse and Alcoholism (NIAAA). (1989, January). Alcohol and trauma. *Alcohol Alert, 3*, 1–4.
National Institute on Alcohol Abuse and Alcoholism (NIAAA). (1990, April). Screening for alcoholism. *Alcohol Alert*, 1–4.
National Institute on Alcohol Abuse and Acoholism (NIAAA). (1991, April). Assessing alcoholism. *Alcohol Alert*, 1–4.
National Institute on Alcohol Abuse and Alcoholism (NIAAA). (1994). *Eighth special report of the U. S. Congress on alcohol and health* (NIH Publication No. 94-3699). Bethesda, MD: National Institute of Health.
National Institute of Health (NIH). (1993). *Drugs and the brain* (NIH Publication No. 93-3057). Bethesda, MD: Author.
Nebelkopf, E. (1981). Holistic programs for the drug addict and alcoholic. *Journal of Psychoactive Drugs, 13*, 345–351.
Neimark, J., Conway, C., & Doskoch, P. (1994, September/October). Back from the drink. *Psychology Today*, 46–53.
Nelson, S., Shellito, J., Mason, C., & Summer, W. R. (1992). Alcohol and bacterial pneumonia. *Alcohol Health & Research World, 16*, 73–80.
Nutt, D. J., & Glue, P. (1990). Neuropharmacological and clinical aspects of alcohol withdrawal. *Annals of Medicine, 22*, 275–281.
Ohims, D. L. (1990). *The disease concept of alcoholism* (pp. 6–18). Hartford, CT: The Institute of Living.
O'Malley, S. S., Jaffe, A., Chang, G., Witte, G., Schottenfeld, R. S., & Rounsaville, B. J. (1992). Naltrexone in the treatment of alcohol dependence: Preliminary findings. In C. A. Naranjo & E. M. Sellers

(Eds.), *Novel pharmacological interventions for alcoholism* (pp. 148–160). New York: Springer-Verlag.

Ortiz, J., Fitzgerald, L. W., Charlton, M., Lane, S., Trevsan, L., Grutart, X., Shoemaker, W., Duman, R. S., & Nestler, E. J. (1995). Biochemical actions of chronic ethanol exposure in the mesolimbic dopamine system. *Synapse, 21*, 289–298.

Oscar-Berman, M. O. (1990). Severe brain dysfunction: Alcoholic Korsakoff's syndrome. *Alcohol Health & Research World, 14*, 120–129.

Oscar-Berman, M. O. (1992, Fall). Alcoholism and asymmetrics of brain function. *Alcohol Health & Research World*, 273–280.

Paffenbarger, R. S., Jr., & Williams, J. L. (1967). Chronic disease in former college students. V. Early precursors of fatal stroke. *American Journal of Public Health, 57*, 1290.

Patel, D. G. (1989). Effects of ethanol on carbohydrate metabolism and implications for the aging alcoholic. *Alcohol Health & Research World, 13*, 240–246.

Porjesz, B., & Begleiter, H. (1995). Event-related potentials and cognitive function in alcoholism. *Alcohol Health & Research World, 19*, 108–112.

Portenoy, R. K., & Payne, R. (1992). Acute and chronic pain. In J. H. Lowinson, P. Ruiz, R. B. Millman, & J. G. Langrod (Eds.), *Substance abuse: A comprehensive textbook* (2nd ed.). Baltimore: Williams & Wilkins.

Porth, C. M. (1994). *Pathophysiology concepts of altered health states* (pp. 847–850, 1180–1182). Phildelphia: J. B. Lippincott.

Rawson, R. A., Obert, J. L., & McCann, M. J. (1991 May/June). Cocaine: Recovery issues. *Addiction & Recovery*, 29–33.

Ray, O. (1983). *Drugs, society, and human behavior* (3rd ed., pp. 183–205). St. Louis, MO: C. V. Mosby.

Ray, O., & Ksir, C. (1993). *Drugs, society, and human behavior* (6th ed.). St. Louis, MO: Mosby-Year Book.

Redfern, T. R., Rees, D., & Owen, R. (1988). The impact of alcohol ingestion on the orthopedic and accident service. *Alcohol & Alcoholism, 23*, 415–419.

Rees, W. D. W., & Turnberg, L. A. (1980). Reappraisal of the effects of aspirin on the stomach. *Lancet, 2*, 410–413.

Reyna, T. M., Hollis, H. W., & Hulsebus, R. C. (1985). Alcohol-related trauma: The surgeon's responsibility. *Annals of Surgery, 201*, 194–197.

Rico, H. (1990). Alcohol and bone disease. *Alcohol & Alcoholism, 25*, 345–352.

Ridley, T. D., & Kordinak, S. T. (1988). Reliability and validity of the quantitative inventory of alcohol disorders (QIAD) and the veracity of self-report by alcoholics. *American Journal of Drugs and Alcohol Abuse, 14*, 263–292.

Ried, L. D., & Hunter, G. A. (1984). Morphine and naloxone modulate intake of ethanol. *Alcohol, 38*, 33–37.

Riggs. S., & Alario, A. J. (1989). Adolescent substance use. In C. Dube, M. Goldstein, & D. C. Lewis (Eds.), *The project ADEPT curriculum for primary care physician training* [Module]. Brown University, Providence, RI.

Rimmele, C. T., Miller, W. R., & Dougher, M. J. (1989). Aversion therapies. In R. K. Hester & W. R. Miller (Eds.), *Handbook of alcoholism treatment approaches: Effective alternatives* (pp. 128–140). New York: Pergamon Press.

Rivara, F. P., Koepsell, T. D., Jurkovich, G. J., Gurney, J. G., & Soderberg, R. (1993). The effects of alcohol abuse on readmission for trauma. *Journal of the Amercian Medical Association, 270*, 1962–1964.

Robertson, N. (1992, February-March). Under the influence. *Modern Maturity, 20*, 26–30, 65.

Roizen, J. (1982). Estimating alcohol involvement in serious events. In National Institute on Alcohol Abuse and Alcoholism (NIAAA), *Alcohol consumption and related problems* (Alcohol and Health Monograph 1, DHHS Publication No. ADM 82-1190, pp. 179–219). Washington, DC: U.S. Government Printing Office.

Roizen, J. (1988). Alcohol and trauma. In N. Giesbrecht, R. Gonzales, M. Grant, E. Osterberg, R. Room, I. Rootman, & L. Towle (Eds.), *Drinking and casualties: Accidents, poisonings, and violence in an international perspective* (pp. 21–69). London: Routledge.

Roselle, G. A. (1992). Alcohol and the immune system. *Alcohol Health & Research World, 16*, 16–22.

Rostenberg, P. O. (1995). *Alcohol and other drug screening of hospitalized trauma patients* (Treatment Improvement Protocol [TIPS] Series 16, DHHS Publication No. SMA 95-3041). Rockville, MD: U.S. Department of Health and Human Services.

Rounsaville, B. J., & Carroll, K. M. (1992). Individual psychotherapy for drug abusers. In J. Lowinson, P. Ruiz, & R. Millman (Eds.), *Substance abuse: A comprehensive textbook* (2nd ed., pp. 496–507). Baltimore: Williams & Wilkins.

Roy, A., DeJong, J., Lamparski, D., George, T., & Linnoila, M. (1991). Depression among alcoholics. *Archives of General Psychiatry, 48*, 428–432.

Rubin, E. (1989). How alcohol damages the body. *Alcohol Health & Research World, 13*, 322–327.

Rubin, E., & Doria, J. (1990). Alcoholic cardiomyopathy. *Alcohol Health & Research World, 14*, 277–284.

Rudorfer, M. W., & Potter, W. Z. (1987). Pharmacokinetics of antidepressants. In H. Y. Meltzer (Ed.), *Psychopharmacology: The third generation of progress* (pp. 1353–1363). New York: Raven Press.

Ryan, C., & Butters, N. (1986). The neuropsychology of alcoholism. In D. Wedding, A. M. Horton, Jr., & J. Webster (Eds.), *The neuropsychology handbook: Behavioral and clinical perspectives* (pp. 376–409). New York: Springer.

Saunders, J. B., Aasland, O. G., Babor, T. F., De La Fuente, J. R., & Grant, M. (1993). Development of the alcohol use disorders identification test (AUDIT): WHO collaborative project on early detection of persons with harmful alcohol consumption. II. *Addiction, 88*, 791–804.

Schmelzer, E. J. (1994). Social work interventions related to substance abuse among spinal cord injury patients: A response to rationalization. *SCI Psychosocial Process, 7*, 117–122.

Schmidt, W., & deLint, J. (1972). Causes of deaths of alcoholics. *Quarterly Journal of Studies on Alcohol, 33*, 171–185.

Schnoll, S. (1986). *Getting help: Treatments for drug abuse*. New York: Chelsea House Publishers.

Schuckit, M. A. (1989). *Drug and alcohol abuse: A clinical guide to diagnosis and treatment* (3rd ed.). New York: Plenum Press.

Sees, K. L. (1991). Pharmacological adjuncts for the treatment of withdrawal syndromes. *Journal of Psychoactive Drugs, 23*, 371–385.

Selzer, M. L. (1971). The Michigan Alcoholism Screening Test: The quest for a new diagnostic instrument. *American Journal of Psychiatry, 127*, 1653–1658.

Selzer, M., Vinokur, A., & van Rooijen, L. (1975). A self-administered Short Michigan Alcohol Screening test (SMAST). *Journal of Studies on Alcohol, 36*, 117–126.

Senay, E. C. (1992). Diagnostic interview and mental status examination. In J. Lowinson, P. Ruiz, & R. Millman (Eds.), *Substance abuse: A comprehensive textbook* (2nd ed., pp. 416–424). Baltimore: Williams & Wilkins.

Seppala, T., Linnoila, M., & Mattila, M. J. (1979). Drugs, alcohol and driving. *Drugs, 17*, 189–408.

Serdula, M., Williamson, D. R., Kendrick, J. S., Anda, R. F., & Beyers, T. (1991). Trends in alcohol consumption by pregnant women: 1985–1988. *Journal of the American Medical Association, 265*, 876–879.

Shaffer, H. J., & Robbins, M. (1995). Psychotherapy for addictive behavior: A stage-change approach to meaning making. In A. M. Washton (Ed.), *Psychotherapy and substance abuse: A practitioner's handbook* (pp. 103–123). New York: Guilford Publications.

Shaw, L., & McMahon, B. (1990). Family-staff conflict in the rehabilitation setting: Causes, consequences and implication. *Brain Injury, 4*, 87–93.

Sheperd, G. M. (1994). *Neurobiology* (3rd ed.). New York: Oxford University Press.

Shlafer, M. (1993). *The nurse pharmacology and drug therapy*. New York: Addison Wesley Nursing.

Shoaf, S. E., & Linnoila, M. (1991). Interaction of ethanol and smoking on the pharmacokinetics and pharmacodynamics of psychotropic medications. *Psychopharmacology Bulletin, 27*, 577–594.

Siegel. S. (1989). Pharmacological conditioning and drug effects. In A. J. Goudie & M. W. Emmett-Oglesby (Eds.), *Psychoactive drugs: Tolerance and sensitization* (pp. 115–180). Clifton, NJ: Humana Press.

Singer, A. (1992). *Effective treatment for drug-involved offenders*. Newton, MA: Education Development Center.

Singh, M. (1990). Ethanol and the pancreas. *Gastroenterology, 98*, 1051–1062.

Skinner, H. A., Holt, S., Schuller, R., Roy, J., & Israell, Y. (1984). Identification of alcohol abuse using laboratory tests and a history of trauma. *Annals of Internal Medicine, 101*, 847–851.

Smith, D. E. (1986). Cocaine-alcohol abuse: Epidemiological, diagnostic and treatment considerations. *Journal of Psychoactive Drugs, 18*, 117–128.

Smith, G., & Krauss, J. (1988). Alcohol and residential, recreational and occupational injuries: A review of the epidemiologic evidence. *Annual Review of Public Health, 9*, 99–121.

Soderstrom, C. A. (1989). Alcohol and trauma: Perspectives and clinical issues. *Advanced Trauma, 4*, 211–240.

Soderstrom, C. A., & Cowley, R. A. (1987). A national alcohol and trauma center survey: Missed opportunities, failures of responsibility. *Archives of Surgery, 122*, 1067–1071.

Soderstrom, C., DuPriest, R., Benner, C., Maekawa, K., & Cowley, R. (1979). Alcohol and roadway trauma: Problems of diagnosis and management. *American Surgery, 45*, 129–135.

Sokol, R. J., Iannaccone, S. T., Bove, K. E., & Heubi, J. E. (1983). Vitamin E deficiency neurologic syndrome during chronic cholestasis: Beneficial effects of early alphatocopherol therapy. *Pediatric Research, 17*, 367.

Sokol, R. J., Martier, S. S., & Ager, J. W. (1989). The T-ACE questions: Practical prenatal detection of risk-drinking. *American Journal of Obstetrics and Gynecology, 160*, 863–870.

Soucy, G. P., Kelly, M. P. P., & Cardenas, E. (1994). A National Institute on Drug Abuse technology transfer package: The addiction severity index for assessing substance-abusing adults. *Substance Abuse, 15*, 13–15.

Sparadeo, F. R., & Gill, D. (1989). Effects of prior alcohol use on head injury recovery. *Journal of Head Trauma Rehabilitation, 4*, 75–82.

Sparadeo, F. R., Strauss, S., & Barth, J. T. (1990). The incidence, impact, and treatment of substance abuse in head trauma rehabilitation. *Journal of Head Trauma Rehabilitation, 5*, 1–8.

Stahl, I. (1992). Yoga as personal development. *Addictions Nursing Network, 4*, 122–125.

Stark, M. J., & Campbell, B. K. (1991). A psychoeducational approach to methadone maintenance treatment: A survey of client reactions. *Journal of Substance Abuse Treatment, 8*, 125–131.

Stewart, J., & Eikelboom, R. (1987). Conditioned drug effects. In L. L. Iverson, S. D. Iverson, & S. H. Snyder (Eds.), *Handbook of psychopharmacology* (Vol. 19, pp. 1–57). New York: Plenum Press.

Stover, S. L., & Fine, P. R. (1986). *Spinal cord injuries: The facts and figures.* Birmingham: University of Alabama at Birmingham.

Swan, K. G. (1989). Recurrent trauma. *Journal of Trauma, 29,* 947.

Swenson, W. M., & Morse, R. M. (1975). The use of a self-administered alcoholism screening test (SAAST) in a medical center. *Mayo Clinic Preceedings, 50,* 204–208.

Swerslow, J. L. (1995). Quiet miracle of the brain. *National Geographic, 186,* 2–41.

Synder, S. H. (Ed.). (1987). *The encyclopedia of psychoactive drugs—Drugs and the brain.* New York: Chelsea House.

Tabakoff, B., Hoffman, P. L., & Peterson, R. C. (1990). Advances in neurochemistry—A leading edge of alcohol research. *Alcohol Health & Research World, 14,* 138–143.

Tarter, R. E., Ott, P. J., & Mezzich, A. C. (1991). Psychometric assessment. In R. J. Frances & S. I. Miller (Eds.), *Clinical textbook of addictive disorders.* New York: Guilford Press.

Ter Reit, G., Kleijnen, J., & Knipschild, P. (1990). A meta-analysis of studies into the effect of acupuncture on addiction. *British Journal of Psychiatry, 40,* 379–382.

Thomas, E. J., Yoshioka, M., & Ager, R. D. (1996). Spouse enabling of alcohol abuse: Conception, assessment, and modification. *Journal of Substance Abuse, 8,* 61–80.

Tollefson, G. D. (1992). Treatment of comorbid generalized anxiety in a recently detoxified alcoholic population with a selective serotonergic drug (buspirone). *Journal of Clinical Psychopharmacology,* 12, 19.

Tortora, G. J., & Anagnostakos, N. P. (1987). *Principles of anatomy and physiology* (5th ed.). New York: Harper & Row Publishers.

Tortora, G. J., & Grabowski, S. R. (1993). *Principles of anatomy and physiology.* New York: HarperCollins College Publishers.

Tsutsumi, R., Leo, M. A., Kim, C.-I., Tsutsumi, M., Lasker, J., Lowe, N., & Lieber, C. S. (1990). Interaction of ethanol with enflurane metabolism and toxicity: Role of P45011E1. Alcoholism: *Clinical and Experimental Research, 14,* 174–179.

Tweed, S. H. (1989). Identifying the alcoholic client. *Nursing Clinics of North America, 24,* 20–32.

Urbano-Marquez, A., Estruch, R., Navarro-Lopez, F., Grau, J. M., Mont, L., & Rubin, E. (1989). The effects of alcoholism on skeletal and cardiac muscle. *New England Journal of Medicine, 320,* 409–415.

Vaillant, F., Schnurr, P., Caron, J., & Gerber, P. (1991). A prospective study of the effects of cigarette smoking and alcohol abuse on mortality. *Journal of General Medicine, 6,* 299–303.

Victor, M., Adams, R. D., & Collins, G. H. (1989). *The Wernicke-Korsakoff syndrome and related neurologic disorders due to alcoholism and malnutrition* (2nd ed.). Philadelphia: F. A. Davis.

Volpicelli, J. R., Davis, M. A., & Olfin, J. E. (1986). Naltrexone blocks the post-shock increase of ethanol consumption. *Life Science*, 841–847.

Volpicelli, J. R., O'Brien, C. P., Alterman, A. I., & Hayashida, M. (1990). Naltrexone and the treatment of alcohol-dependence: Initial observations. In L. D. Reid (Ed.), *Opioids, bulimia and alcohol abuse and alcoholism* (pp. 195–214). New York: Springer-Verlag.

Walinder, J., Balldin, J., Bokstrom, K., Karlsson, I., & Lundstrom, B. (1981). Clonidine suppression of the alcohol withdrawal syndrome. *Drug and Alcohol Dependence, 8*, 345–348.

Wallace, P., & Haines, A. (1985). The use of a questionnaire in general practice to increase the recognition of patients' excessive alcohol consumption. *British Medical Journal, 290*, 1949–1593.

Waller, P. F., Hansen, A. R., & Stewart, J. R. (1989, October). *The potentiating effects of alcohol on injury: A clinical study.* Paper presented at the Annual Meeting of the Association for Advancement of Automotive Medicine, Baltimore, MD.

Washton, A. M. (1988). Nonpharmacologic treatment of cocaine abuse. *Psychiatric Clinics of North America, 9*, 563–571.

Weil, A. (1990). *Natural health, natural medicine—A comprehensive manual for wellness & self care.* Boston: Houghton Mifflin.

Wen, H. L., & Cheung, S. Y. C. (1973). Treatment of drug addiction by acupuncture and electrical stimulation. *Asian Journal of Medicine, 9*, 138.

Wesson, D. R., & Ling, W. (1991, October/December). Medications in the treatment of addictive disease. *Journal of Psychoactive Drugs, 23*, 365–370.

Whitehead, P. C. (1978). Acupuncture in the treatment of addiction: A review and analysis. *International Journal of the Addictions, 13*, 1–16.

Whitfield, C. C. (1984). Co-alcoholism: Recognizing a treatable illness. *Family and Community Health, 7*, 16–25.

Wilkens, J. N., & Gorelick, D. A. (1986). Clinical neuroendocrinology and neuropharmacology of alcohol withdrawal. In M. Galanter (Ed.), *Recent developments in alcoholism* (Vol. 4, pp. 241–263). New York: Plenum Press.

Williams, G., III. (1996). The healing power of prayer. *McCalls*, 86–89.

Williams, M. (1984). Alcohol and the elderly. *Alcohol Health & Research World, 8*, 3–9, 52.

Winters, K. C., & Zenilman, J. M. (1994). *Simple screening instruments for outreach for alcohol and other drug abuse and infectious diseases* (Treatment Improvement Protocol [TIPS] Series 11, DHHS Publication No. SMA 94–2094). Rockville, MD: U.S. Department of Health and Human Services.

Wolf, P. A., Kannel, W. B., & Verter, J. (1983). Current status of risk factors for stroke. *Neurology Clinic, 10*, 177–191.

Woody, G. E., McLellan, A. T., Luborsky, L., & O'Brien, C. P. (1985). Sociopathy and psychotherapy outcome. *Archives of General Psychiatry, 42*, 1081–1086.

Woody, G. E., McLellan, A. T., Luborsky, L., & O'Brien, C. P. (1990). Psychotherapy and counseling for methadone-maintained opiate addicts: Results of research studies. In L. S. Oken & J. D. Blaine (Eds.), *Psychotherapy and counseling in the treatment of drug abuse* (National Institute on Drug Abuse [NIDA] Research Monograph Series 104, NIH Publication No. 94-3716, pp. 9–23). Washington, DC: U.S. Government Printing Office.

Zakhari, S. (1991). Vulnerability to cardiac disease. In M. Galanter (Ed.), *Recent developments in alcoholism* (Vol. 9, pp. 225–262). New York: Plenum Press.

Zilm, D. H., Jacob, M. S., MacLeod, S. M., Sellers, E. M., & Ti, T. Y. (1980). Propranolol and chlordiazepoxide effects on cardiac arrhymias during alcohol withdrawal. *Alcoholism: Clinical and Experimental Research, 4*, 400–405.

Zimberg, S. (1985). Treating the older alcoholic. *Geriatric Medicine Today, 4*, 68–70, 76–77.

Zweben, A., Pearlman, S., & Li, S. (1988). A comparison of brief advice and conjoint therapy in the treatment of alcohol abuse: The results of the Marital Systems study. *British Journal of Addiction, 83*, 899–916.

Zweben, J. E. (1993). Review of clinical issues. In Center for Substance Abuse Treatment (CSAT), *State methadone treatment guidelines*, (Treatment Improvement Protocol [TIP] Series No. 1, DHHS Publication No. SMA 93–1991, pp. 25–32). Rockville, MD: U.S. Department of Health and Human Services.

Zweben, J. E., & O'Connell, K. (1992). Strategies for breaking marijuana dependence. *Journal of Psychoactive Drugs, 24*, 165–171.

INDEX

E

F

L

M

N

S

T